Pound-a-Day
Rapid Weight Loss™

The Easiest Weight You'll Ever Lose While Achieving Your Best Health Ever!

SECOND EDITION

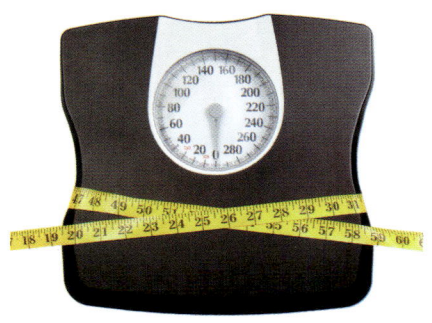

by Madison Cavanaugh

Pound-a-Day Rapid Weight Loss™: The Easiest Weight You'll Ever Lose While Achieving Your Best Health Ever! *Second Edition*

Copyright © 2023 Think-Outside-the-Book, Inc.

No part of this publication may be reproduced, stored in a retrieval system or transmitted in any form or by any means, electronic, mechanical, photocopying, recording or otherwise without the written permission of the publisher.

Publisher:
Think-Outside-the-Book, Inc.
Summerlin, Nevada 89117

Disclaimer: The entire contents of this book are based upon research conducted by the author, unless otherwise noted. The publisher, the author, the distributors and bookstores present this information for educational purposes only. This information is not intended to diagnose or prescribe for medical or psychological conditions or to claim to prevent, treat, mitigate or cure such conditions. The author and the publisher are not making an attempt to recommend specific products as treatment of disease. In presenting this information, no attempt is being made to provide diagnosis, care, treatment or rehabilitation of individuals, or apply medical, mental health or human development principles, to provide diagnosing, treating, operating or prescribing for any human disease, pain, injury, deformity or physical condition. The information contained herein is not intended to replace a one-on-one relationship with a doctor or qualified health care professional. Therefore, the reader should be made aware that this information is not intended as medical advice, but rather a sharing of knowledge and information from the research and experience of the author. The publisher and the author encourage you to make your own health care decisions based upon your research and in partnership with a qualified health care professional. You and only you are responsible if you choose to do anything based on what you read.

Table of Contents

Author's Introduction to the Second Edition of Pound-a-Day Rapid Weight Loss™ 1

Chapter One
The Pound-a-Day Rapid Weight Loss™ Program – in a Nutshell

The easiest weight you'll ever lose – the last weight loss program you'll ever try 7

Chapter Two
Why the Program Works: The 5 Most Effective Weight Loss Strategies in One 15

Green Smoothie: *The 3-minute breakfast that may be the "Healthiest Meal in the World!"* 15

Glucomannan (Konjac Root): *Flush up to 25% of calories consumed; 78% of each pound lost is pure body fat* 20

The "Self-Indulgent Meal of the Day": *Eat any food you want – with just one tiny twist (hara hachi bu) that accelerates weight loss* 22

Pu-Erh Tea: *Scientifically proven to shrink fat cells, increase metabolism, help shed water weight, and prevent the body from turning the food you eat into fat* 27

Organic Chia Seeds: *The best overall weight control and appetite control for losing one pound a day* 30

Chapter Three
Fast Track Your Way to Even Faster Weight Loss

Lose a dress or pant size in one week 37

Chapter Four
Customize the Pound-a-Day Rapid Weight Loss™ Program for <u>Your</u> Specific Lifestyle

Why you can "cheat" any day of the week and still lose weight! 49

Chapter Five
28 Days of Nutritionally Balanced Recipes

Delicious, kitchen-tested recipes that support your Pound-a-Day weight loss goal 55

Chapter Six
Your Green Smoothie Recipes 99

Chapter Seven
The 1-Minute Mindset Technique

Scientifically "rewire your brain" to get rid of food cravings, compulsive eating habits and emotional factors that are obstacles to losing weight 109

Chapter Eight
The 20-Second Workout

The minimum effective dose of exercise which will give you a lean, firm, toned and metabolically efficient body 129

Recommended Websites and Resources 161

Author's Introduction to the Second Edition of the Pound-a-Day Rapid Weight Loss™

How many times have you tried to lose weight in the past 12 months? If you're like the average dieter, you probably try 4 or 5 different times every year, don't you?

But sadly ... with every try, you've *failed* to keep the weight off, haven't you?

I'm certain that *some* weight loss programs may have enabled you to lose weight <u>initially</u> -- but soon thereafter, like a cruel joke, the weight has crept back on, hasn't it? And you often end up weighing more than you did before you tried to lose weight.

Yes, the weight loss "hamster wheel" can be so frustrating -- especially if you're eating well, exercising, and using all the effort and will power you can muster ... but the darned weight just won't come off or stay off!

How has your string of failures made you feel? Trying and failing over and over again is *painful*, isn't it?

I know. I've been in your shoes.

I was naturally slim when I was in my teens and early twenties, but after I reached the age of thirty, I began to pile on the excess weight. At first, it was just a few unwanted pounds ... but before long, it was 5 pounds, then 10, 12, and 15 pounds of stubborn weight that simply wouldn't come off permanently, no matter how many hours I spent working out or whatever diet I tried. But when I tipped the scale at 23 pounds over my normal weight, that's when I began to panic!

Twenty-three pounds might not seem like a lot of excess weight to most people, but on a small-boned, petite woman like myself, twenty pounds overweight put my Body Mass Index (BMI) at a level that was borderline obese! I had gone up 3 dress sizes, could no longer fit into any of my clothes, and had to buy a new wardrobe to fit my progressively increasing body circumference!

So I know the pain of failing all too well. Just like you, I've tried diet after diet ... fat-burning pills, exercise gadgets, grueling workouts -- and I've bought just about everything on the Internet, TV or radio that promised to make me lose weight.

Every time I failed to keep the weight off, I felt *utterly defeated* and, worst of all ... powerless. And these repeated failures made me feel powerless over <u>everything else</u> in my life. If I couldn't even control my weight, how could I possibly achieve anything, least of all my dreams?

Have you felt the same pain?

Since you're reading this book, I'm sure you have felt the same pain ... and you continue to feel that pain every day.

And that's why I'm going to tell you about my weight loss journey -- and how I came to develop the Pound-a-Day Rapid Weight Loss program that enables average people like you and me to achieve permanent weight loss—even when nothing else has worked before. This has literally changed my life and the lives of countless people with whom I shared this one-of-a-kind program.

Back in 2014, when the concept of Pound-a-Day Rapid Weight Loss first came into my purview, it enabled me to easily lose the 23 pounds of excess weight that I had accumulated over the previous 25 years. In a matter of weeks, I was able to lose a combined 8" in circumference, and got back to the dress size I haven't been able to fit into for 25 years. As of the time of this writing, I've kept the weight off and have maintained my ideal weight for 9 years ... and counting.

So I was convinced then--as I am now--that the Pound-a-Day Rapid Weight Loss program works like nothing else in the weight loss industry! The program spawned thousands of followers who sent in countless testimonials reporting how they easily shed pounds on the program -- and that it was "the easiest weight they ever lost."

Clinically Obese Man Loses 45 Pounds

"I've been in denial for a very long time. I knew I was overweight, but kept insisting that I only needed to lose 15 to 20 pounds. But I was actually more than 50 pounds overweight. My wife checked the charts and discovered that based on my height and age, I was actually clinically obese! I've tried to lose weight for as long as I can remember -- and I've tried everything, but nothing worked.

"I found out about Pound-a-Day Rapid Weight Loss last December, and I got on the program right away. I lost so many pounds in the first week, and I got excited! I continued losing weight until I lost over 45 pounds, and now I'm no longer obese but have crossed over to the Healthy Weight range! People who hadn't seen me in months could hardly recognize me. This is truly the ONLY thing that has ever worked for me -- and it's the easiest weight I've ever lost!" -- Ron F., Tracy, California

So what exactly is Pound-a-Day Rapid Weight Loss?

Pound-a-Day Rapid Weight Loss is a doctor-endorsed eating strategy that combines 5 of the most effective, scientifically proven weight loss strategies into one powerful system that enables you to easily lose up to a pound a day of excess weight in a _healthy manner_. Unlike the Keto diet, or the Mediterranean, Sonoma, Paleo, Atkins, Scarsdale, Low-Carb, South Beach, or Dukan diets you may have tried before, the Pound-a-Day Rapid Weight Loss program is _not a diet_ at all. It is the only program that ...

- allows you to eat your favorite foods (no meal plan or restrictive diet)
- does not require you to count calories or measure the amount of food you consume
- enables you to lose weight consistently -- without disrupting your lifestyle or your daily activities
- is so simple and easy to follow that you'll want to stick to it ... for life!
- is suitable for men and women of all ages, body types and sizes
- enables you to lose weight -- but more importantly, keep the weight off effortlessly,
- is so effective that it will be "**the last weight loss program you'll ever try**"

And best of all, the 3 supplements that are key to the effectiveness of the Pound-a-Day Rapid Weight Loss program (glucomannan capsules 2000mg, organic chia seeds and pu-erh tea), are all available online at www.OnePoundADay.com and other online retailers -- and cost less than 50 cents a day!

In addition to the brilliant eating strategy, this second edition of the Pound-a-Day Rapid Weight Loss program also includes a 1-minute mindset technique that scientifically "rewires your brain" to help you get rid of food cravings, compulsive eating habits, and emotional factors that might sabotage your weight loss efforts. It enables you to overcome your deep-seated *mental*, *emotional* and *psychological* obstacles and pitfalls to losing weight, thereby making it impossible for you to fail. Since it takes only a minute, it's easy to incorporate into your daily activities.

So now that you know you can lose a pound of unwanted weight per day on the Pound-a-Day Rapid Weight Loss program, what comes next?

You probably know people who have lost a lot of weight--or some who have never been overweight to begin with--but they still don't have what you would consider to be an awesome body. That's because their bodies—slim though they may be—lack tone, firmness and definition. That is exactly why this book includes the 20-second workout which will enable you to achieve a lean, toned, firm and well-defined body.

The 20-second workout presented in Chapter 8 is a modified version of the traditional high-intensity interval training (HIIT) workout -- but each exercise takes only 20 seconds to do.

Why 20 seconds?

Because the **minimum effective dose of exercise** you can do -- and still see results -- is **20 seconds**. It takes as little as 20 seconds per muscle group to experience a change in your physique.

When you engage one muscle group with a 20-second high-intensity contraction, your muscles become toned (instead of wasting away from disuse). This makes your body more metabolically efficient, and turns your body into a fat-burning furnace. Cycling through ten of the 20-second exercises that target various muscle groups takes only 5½ minutes, 3 times a week. Who doesn't have 5½ minutes to sculpt a perfectly toned body?

To recap, the rapid weight Loss program that you will discover in this book will enable you to lose a pound of unwanted weight per day. The 1-minute mindset technique will rewire your brain to get rid of food cravings, compulsive eating habits, and enable you to overcome your *mental, emotional* and *psychological* obstacles to losing weight. And the 20-second workout will give you a lean, firm, toned and metabolically efficient body.

Whether you want to lose 30 to 50 pounds or more -- or you just want to get rid of those last 5 to 10 pounds of stubborn weight -- the *Pound-a-Day Rapid Weight Loss* program will enable you to finally get off the yo-yo dieting cycle of insanity, and set you on the fast track to achieving your goal.

Chapter One

The Pound-a-Day Rapid Weight Loss™ Program – in a Nutshell

The easiest weight you'll ever lose – the last weight loss program you'll ever try

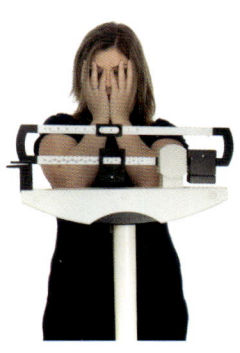

How many weight loss programs are there in the world? The actual count is unknown, but one thing is for certain: There are more weight loss programs and products available on the market today than at any other time in history.

And yet, there are more overweight and obese people than ever before.

Why is that? Does it mean that none of the weight loss programs or products are effective? No, not at all.

The fact is, most weight loss programs are **effective** … *at first*. They all work to some degree, and people who try them get various levels of success. But whenever people embark on a weight loss program, over time, one—or more—of the following five things happens:

- They find that the weight loss program is **not sustainable**—oftentimes, it's too restrictive for them to stay on it for the rest of their lives. So they aren't able to stick to the program for more than a few weeks or months—and the weight they lost initially is gained back.

- They begin to feel **deprived** because their weight loss program doesn't allow them to eat the food they want to eat or have the lifestyle they want to have. So they eventually quit, and slide back into their old eating habits—and often gain back the pounds they lost, usually more than they lost.

- They find that even though their weight loss program does make them lose weight, it has **undesirable effects on their health**—such as diminished mental performance, headaches and muscle weakness (from low-carb diets) … heart palpitations or jitters (from fat burners and stimulants) … loss of energy and low blood sugar (from caloric restrictions) ... loss of brain energy and shaky feeling (from restricted food intake) ... fatigue and loss of skin elasticity (from low-fat or zero-fat diets) ... and low quality of health from yo-yo dieting. The keto diet, for instance, carries a plethora of adverse health effects. It may lead to high cholesterol and an increased risk of heart disease due to unrestricted consumption of saturated fat. Keto may also lead to serious muscle loss; put stress on the kidneys and cause kidney stones; cause dangerously low blood sugar (which is risky for diabetics); cause bowel problems, such as constipation; may lead to nutrient deficiencies; may cause digestive issues and changes in gut bacteria, and increase your risk of chronic diseases, such as heart disease or cancer.

- Their **weight loss program stops working**—most weight loss programs don't have long-term efficacy. For example, after six months, the efficacy of low-carbohydrate diets diminishes, and people begin to regain weight.

- The weight loss program is usually **not balanced** from a health standpoint—low-carb diets don't include enough fruits, vegetables and whole grains for long-term health ... meal replacement powders and protein bars are chock-full of unhealthy hydrogenated oil, fake fats and trans fatty acids ... and many weight loss plans cause a wide array of health problems.

Is it any wonder why the world is still filled with overweight people? About 41.9% of the people in America are obese, according to the Centers for Disease Control and Prevention. Obesity is defined as roughly 35 pounds over a healthy weight. Approximately 17.1% of U.S. adults aged 20 and over are on a special diet on any given day -- which means that an estimated 108 million people are on diets in the United States alone, according to the ABC network's *20/20*.

Dieters typically make **four to five attempts to lose weight per year**. But when it comes to weight loss, there is no truer maxim than this:

**"The ONLY diet that works is
the one you can stick to."**

Now, with the advent of the Pound-a-Day Rapid Weight Loss program, you've finally found the **ultimate eating strategy** -- *not a diet* -- that you can easily stick to for life. That's why this will be the last weight loss attempt you'll ever make—because you will lose weight permanently this time.

> **Susan Lost 27 Pounds in 30 Days!**
>
> "I gained so much weight after overeating during the Christmas holidays and going on a 7-day cruise in February where I ate everything in sight. I thought I probably gained 10 pounds, but when I got on the weighing scale at the beginning of March, I was horrified to see that I was 25 pounds overweight! It was the heaviest I've ever been in my life. I got on the intermittent fasting diet right away and did a yoga workout 3X a week, but only managed to lose 2 pounds. I heard about the Pound-A-Day weight loss progam, and I got started on March 31. I lost 2.7 pounds in 3 days, and became a believer. By April 30, I had lost 27 pounds! When I attended my niece's wedding in May, all my relatives begged to know what I had done to lose so much weight so fast! I told them about Pound-a-Day, and 7 of them got started on the program the following week!" -- Susan H., St. George, Utah

What is the Pound-a-Day Rapid Weight Loss program, and why is it different from any other weight loss program that has ever been developed?

It is a doctor-endorsed eating strategy that **combines five of the most effective, scientifically proven weight loss strategies** which, when examined individually, work quite well—but when all five are combined, they turn into one powerful program that allows you **lose one pound of excess weight per day ... eat the foods you love ... never go on a "diet" ... achieve your ideal weight with the greatest of ease** ... while **making yourself healthier than you've ever been.**

Best of all, the program is so easy-to-follow and sustainable that you'll want to make it your health regimen for life.

> **Mother of Two Kids Loses 17 Pounds in One Month!**
>
> "I got on the Pound-A-Day Rapid Weight Loss program in the first week of January after the holidays were behind us. I found it easy to follow -- even though I have 2 young kids who I have to feed all day long, and so I'm always exposed to their food and snacks.
>
> "It was so easy to stick to the program -- and in about a month, I lost 17 pounds, which is a LOT of weight for me since I'm only 5'1. And I was finally able to fit into my skinny jeans that I had not been able to wear since before I got pregnant with my first child! I was beyond thrilled!" -- Cassandra S., Mountain House, California

The combination of the five weight loss strategies is so unique and easy to follow. Here's the simple Pound-a-Day Rapid Weight Loss plan in a nutshell:

1) **Hydrate Yourself:**
Take a 16-oz glass of water upon waking up in the morning.

2) **Green Smoothie:**
One hour after taking the water, have a green smoothie consisting of 60% fruits and 40% green leafy vegetables (preferably organic). This is one of the healthiest meals one can have that also supports weight loss —and it only takes three minutes to make.

Note: Green smoothie recipes (including those that facilitate fat-burning and accelerate weight loss) can be found in Chapter Six.

3) **Glucomannan (Konjac Root):**
Thirty minutes before lunch, take 2 to 4 capsules of glucomannan (from Konjac Root, totaling 2000mg or more) with at least 8 ounces of water.

Note: In a double-blind study, not only did people taking this dietary supplement in this exact dosage lose weight, but **78% of each pound lost was pure body fat**.

4) **"Self-Indulgent Meal of the Day":**
Thirty minutes after taking the glucomannan capsules, have your "self-indulgent meal of the day." In this meal, you can eat anything you want (within reason), but **eat only until you are 80% full**.

Note: Eating until you're 80% full is an Okinawan practice that accelerates weight loss and enhances health. The amazing info on this weight loss strategy, and useful tips for helping you eat until you're only 80% full, can be found in Chapter Two.

You will never starve or feel deprived on this program because you get to eat a hearty lunch of your choice. For accelerated weight loss, you can choose the healthier versions of popular foods like pizza, burgers, fries, Mac 'n Cheese, hotdogs, meatloaf—by considering the delicious, kitchen-tested recipes found in Chapter Five.

5) **Organic Pu-Erh Tea:**
Immediately after lunch, take two cups of **organic pu-erh tea**.

Note: Aged pu-erh tea is scientifically proven to shrink fat cells, increase metabolism, help shed water weight, and prevent your body from turning the food you eat into fat. Celebrities like Victoria Beckham, Joss Stone and many others use pu-erh tea to lose weight fast.

6) **Optional Mid-Afternoon Snack:**
You can choose from among a number of healthy snack options, but only if you get hungry in the mid-afternoon. It is unlikely to get hungry because the pu-erh tea also tends to suppress cravings.

Note: For a list of healthy, non-fattening snacks that actually support weight loss, see Chapter Five.

7) **Organic Chia Seed Drink:**
Instead of dinner, have a 16-oz glass of water with a full scoop (13 grams) or 2 tablespoons of organic chia seeds. Let the mixture sit for a few minutes until thickened, and stir before drinking. Make sure to drink this before 7:00 PM.

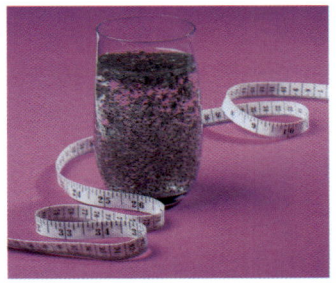

Note: After being in your digestive system for 30 minutes, the organic chia seeds form a highly viscous gel. The seeds' unique fiber coating absorbs the water and forms a gelatinous mass that the body perceives as a big chunk of food, thereby giving the feeling of fullness while also providing extraordinary nutrition that surpasses that of an average meal.

Dr. Bob Arnot, bestselling author and world-renowned Emmy award winning medical correspondent, said he easily lost 1 pound a day by using a scoop (13 grams) of organic chia seeds—and declared it as "the best overall weight control and appetite control" that he's ever found.

Optional: In order to boost the nutritional content of the chia seed evening drink, you can add a scoop of green superfood powder (see the *Resources* section of this book for information on the most nutrient-dense superfood powder blends).

And that's the Pound-a-Day Rapid Weight Loss standard program in a nutshell.

Dr. Brenda Vanta is a medical doctor specialized in nutrition and integrative medicine. She has written more than 800 research-based articles on the subject of diets, nutrients and herbs for various diseases. Upon reviewing the Pound-a-Day Rapid Weight Loss program, she described it as follows:

> "I have reviewed countless diet plans, and found that most of them are not healthy—or they simply don't work on a long-term basis. The Pound-a-Day Rapid Weight Loss program, however, is a superbly designed program for losing weight in a healthy and effective way. The components of the program are awesome for their micronutrient content, the high-quality dietary fiber, low carbohydrates and healthy fats, including healthy essential fatty acids. The program also provides outstanding strategies for losing weight and keeping the weight off in a healthy manner, while boosting your energy levels. The author did research the recommended supplements. I am personally a big fan of the 3 supplements. It is a brilliant program—use it and you'll know why I endorse it."

The beauty of this program is that you can customize it to suit your specific lifestyle and preferences—and still lose a pound a day or more.

If you're an active person, for instance, who works out at the gym in the afternoon, your body might require an actual meal (dinner) after your workout because the chia seed drink may not be something you'd like to have for dinner. If so, there's a customized plan for you. Or if you're a busy mother of young children, for example, and you need to synchronize your meal times with those of your kids, you can customize the plan to work with your busy schedule. If you're the kind of person who simply needs to have 3 square meals a day, you can also customize the plan to your liking.

There are so many ways to customize the plan to suit your needs, your preferences, your body type, and your lifestyle—without compromising the weight loss and health results that you get from the program. In fact, you can "cheat" on the standard Pound-a-Day Rapid Weight Loss program any day of the week—and as many times as you have to—and still lose weight. This is what Pound-a-Day Rapid Weight Loss users love about the program. It's so flexible and not as stringent as the other weight loss programs tend to be.

You'll never feel like you're on a diet (because you're <u>not</u>), and the program is so "forgiving" when you can't stick strictly to the guidelines. This is also why the Pound- A-Day Rapid Weight Loss program is quite sustainable as a lifestyle, and therefore supports long-term weight maintenance. The pounds you lose won't come back whether you're on the standard program or a customized version of the program.

To see how you can customize the Pound-a-Day Rapid Weight Loss program for your lifestyle, see Chapter Four.

The 3 supplements that you'll need for the Pound-a-Day Rapid Weight Loss program (glucomannan capsules 2000mg, organic chia seeds and pu-erh tea), are all available online at www.OnePoundADay.com. See *Recommended Websites and Resources* for other recommended brands. All three will cost you less than $0.49 per day, depending on where you purchase them. Therefore, at a cost of only $15.00 a month, you could conceivably lose 30 pounds in 30 days!

Sacramento Woman Lost 6 Inches of Belly Fat and 22 Pounds in 4 Weeks!

"I lost 22 pounds in just over 4 weeks -- even though I "cheated" on the program several times a week. I also lost 3.5 inches off my waistline, 6 inches off my belly, and a total of 16 inches off my upper body. Pound-a-Day is the only weight loss program that has worked consistently for me." -- J. Andrews, Sacramento, California

Chapter Two

Why the Program Works:
The 5 Most Effective Weight Loss Strategies in One

The Pound-a-Day Rapid Weight Loss program is the first program that combines the "Fantastic Fivesome" of weight loss strategies into one easy plan. So unique is this doctor-endorsed combination that a trademark and Provisional Patent has been filed for it with the U.S. Patent Office.

When you read the details of each of the components that make up the Pound-a-Day Rapid Weight Loss program, its power becomes self-evident, and you'll realize why it will help you finally lose all your unwanted weight, one pound a day. Although many health advocates insist that losing a pound a day is quite drastic, the balanced nutritional profile of all the 5 components combined supports optimum health despite the rapid weight loss.

You may find that even after you've reached your ideal weight, you will want to stay on the program as part of your healthy lifestyle.

The 5 powerhouse components of the Pound-a-Day Rapid Weight Loss program are as follows:

Green Smoothie

The 3-Minute Breakfast that may be the "Healthiest Meal in the World"

There is one simple daily habit that could not only enable you to easily lose excess weight, but also supercharge your energy, detoxify your body, slow down your aging process, prevent practically any chronic disease, and support the healthy functioning of your body. And best of all, it tastes so good.

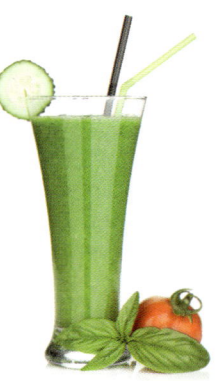

The simple daily habit is that of drinking green smoothies.

Green smoothies are a type of healthy shake made by blending together fruits (such as bananas, apples, strawberries, blueberries, mangoes, pears—fresh or frozen) with green raw leafy vegetables, such as spinach, kale, Swiss chard, collard greens, celery, or broccoli, plus water or ice.

To strike a balance of nutrition and flavor, the typical ratio in a green smoothie is about 60% fruit to 40% leafy greens (preferably organic). Some people add almond milk to make the smoothie a bit creamier.

A green smoothie is regarded by many as the healthiest meal on earth. And although most recipes end up looking like unappetizing liquefied spinach, green smoothies are actually delicious—and enjoyed by adults and children alike—especially when they include your favorite fruits in season.

There's no better way to get the ball rolling on the Pound-a-Day Rapid Weight Loss program each morning than with a green smoothie breakfast—one hour after taking a tall glass of water. The average green smoothie takes approximately 3 to 5 minutes to prepare and consume, so it's a convenient health drink for busy people, and an excellent replacement for the standard breakfast of bacon and eggs or coffee and a Danish pastry.

Why Green Smoothies are an Excellent Breakfast

Contrary to popular belief, breakfast need not be the biggest meal of the day. Although breakfast must necessarily be nutritious in order to sustain you through the morning hours, it should not consist of empty foods that do nothing but fill your stomach.

Most people think a hearty breakfast consists of either eggs and bacon (or sausage or ham) with a slice of buttered toast ... a bowl of cereal with milk ... an omelet ... a doughnut, a bagel with cream cheese, or a Danish pastry—with coffee, tea or orange juice.

These types of meals are not ideal food choices for breakfast.

Here's why: The word *breakfast* literally refers to breaking the fasting period of the prior night. Since your body's "mini-hibernation" slowed down your metabolism for several hours, the last thing you want to do is consume a huge breakfast that will shock your digestive system when it's unprepared to take on the load just yet. If you've ever been on any type of fast that lasts a few days, for instance, all the health experts warn you against consuming too much food at the end of your fast. The body needs time to get acclimatized to eating again, and it's always advisable to increase food intake gradually.

Likewise, since breakfast essentially means "breaking a fast" that lasted several nighttime hours, you must also reach for a first meal that is nutritious—without shocking the digestive system.

Green smoothies are a gradual way to ease the body into digesting food again. And because the fruits and vegetables in a green smoothie are pre-digested in the blender, the body doesn't have to work too hard to digest the food.

Delicious kitchen-tested green smoothie recipes can be found in Chapter Six.

How Green Smoothies Help You Lose Weight

A green smoothie is a low-calorie beverage that is satisfying and nourishing, and one that also curbs cravings you might have for unhealthy food items. It's also an excellent way for you to sneak a large amount of fruits and vegetables—and fiber!—into your diet that you normally wouldn't be able to consume in your regular meals.

If you're a parent of young children or teenagers, green smoothies are also an ideal breakfast to serve your kids because the delicious taste of the smoothie disguises the fact that it's actually good for their health.

Many health practitioners claim that when you include 5 fruits and 3 vegetables into your diet every day, it's almost impossible to develop a chronic disease. The human body benefits tremendously from the optimum nutrition of fruits and vegetables that are in a green smoothie.

My favorite green smoothie recipe is as follows:

> **Banana-Berries-Spinach-Kale (serves 2):**
>
> 2 bananas
>
> ½ cup frozen strawberries
>
> ½ cup frozen blueberries
>
> A handful of shredded kale leaves
>
> 1 bag (6 ounces) of baby spinach
> (from Trader Joe's or supermarket)
>
> 2 cups of pure or filtered water
>
> Optional: A handful of dried goji berries
>
> 2 scoops of a superfood powder blend
> (to boost nutritional content)

Why Have a Green Smoothie Instead of a Fruit/Vegetable Juice?

A juicer extracts the juice of fruits and vegetables, but discards the pulp into the waste chamber of the extractor. Even when one uses a masticating juicer that squeezes every drop of juice from the produce—leaving only dry pulp—that pulp, which is often discarded, contains one of the main health benefits of fruit and vegetable consumption, that is, fiber. On the other hand, blending liquefies the whole fruit or vegetable, and keeps the fiber in the blend instead of discarding it.

Many nutritionists believe that drinking juices extracted from vegetables with high sugar content (such a carrots) or from sweet fruits (such as dates, apples, lychees and bananas) will spike the body's insulin levels, affect blood sugar levels and lead to an increased risk of developing diabetes and cardiovascular disease. That's not the case with *blended fruits and vegetables*. That's because they contain fiber, which slows down the release of natural sugars into the bloodstream.

High-powered blenders like Blendtec and Vita-Mix are able to break down the cell walls of the fruits and vegetables, thereby releasing all the nutrients that the body can readily absorb.

Another advantage of blending is that the green smoothies retain their freshness longer than juices. Although it's always best to consume smoothies as soon as they're blended, they can be refrigerated for up to a few days. Juices, however, begin oxidizing as soon as the juice has been prepared, and they should therefore, be consumed immediately. Otherwise, the juice's nutritional content significantly deteriorates.

> Resist the temptation of making a green smoothie by using store-bought fruit juices blended with green leafy vegetables. Although it might seem like a convenient way to shortcut the process of making green smoothies, commercially available fruit juices actually top the list of beverages that one must NOT consume if one needs to lose weight. Most commonly consumed juice products—whether bottled or cartoned—contain high-fructose corn syrup (HFCS), which is counterproductive to weight loss and also harmful to one's health.
>
> Furthermore, whether a store-bought fruit juice contains HFCS or not, it usually has a significant fructose content. Fructose is a fruit sugar that naturally occurs in fruits, plants and honey. Excess fructose consumption is known to be associated with risk for metabolic disease. Fructose content in fruit juices is often difficult to detect because of the unlabeled quantity of fructose in commercial beverages.

One of the most stunning success stories of extreme weight loss is that of Clent Manich. *The Green Smoothie Phenomenon* book tells the story of this former Costco employee from Medford, Oregon. A few years ago, he weighed 447 pounds. He had struggled with excess weight all his life, and before long, he developed acute pancreatitis. He also suffered from Type II diabetes, with blood sugar over 600, and his triglycerides were over 6,000! He was what doctors would call "a ticking time bomb."

It was Dr. Donato, a Gerson therapy health practitioner who taught Clent how he could turn his health around and save himself from certain death. Clent followed Doctor Donato's advice, which included drinking green smoothies every day. In just three weeks, Clent's health made a remarkable 180-degree turnaround. He was able to overcome his diabetes, and was completely off insulin and all his medications! In 14 weeks, he lost 100 pounds—he eventually dropped 226 pounds in one year, and has never regained the weight.

How did he accomplish such extreme weight loss? Clent started each day by making a gallon of green smoothie made of blended fruits and vegetables. He drank it throughout the day—every two to three hours. Although Clent's previous diets always made him feel hungry and weak, the green smoothies gave him abundant energy and helped eliminate his food cravings, so he was never hungry.

Clent is not alone in his weight loss triumph. Literally tens of thousands of people from all over the world have lost a tremendous amount of weight by incorporating a green smoothie or two into their daily diet.

Clent's story serves to underscore the power of green smoothies in achieving weight loss success. But it doesn't mean you're going to have to drink a gallon of green smoothies a day like Clent did. Just one delicious green smoothie for breakfast is all you need because there are four other components in Pound-A-Day Rapid Weight Loss program that you'll be easily adopting for the rest of the day.

The green smoothie recipes presented in Chapter Six, many of which facilitate fat-burning and weight loss, will provide you with a variety of flavors that will excite your taste buds. Using the typical ratio of a green smoothie (about 60% fruit to 40% leafy greens), you can also create recipes of your own to suit your taste, and to include fruits that are in season.

The essential appliance you'll need to blend your green smoothies together is a commercial-grade blender, such as Vita-Mix or Blendtec. Although a regular blender would suffice in the beginning, you may find that it doesn't have the sufficient power to liquefy or emulsify fibrous vegetables and hard fruits.

If the price of a brand new Vita-Mix or Blendtec blender is beyond your budget, you may choose to buy a certified refurbished Blendtec or Vita-Mix at a greatly reduced price. (Simply type the keywords "refurbished Blendtec" or "refurbished Vitamix" into the Amazon.com or eBay.com search box and you're likely to find one for sale.). Owning a Blendtec or Vita-Mix (whether brand new or refurbished) is one of the best health investments you'll ever make, and will help you lose weight, too.

Glucomannan (Konjac Root)

*Flush up to 25% of calories consumed;
78% of each pound lost is pure body fat*

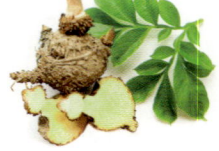

Konnyaku is a traditional Japanese food made from the corm (i.e., the short, thick food-storing underground stem) of the konnyaku potato or konjac plant (*Amorphophallus konjac*), also known as the Devil's Tongue plant. Konnyaku potatoes are cultivated for food only in Japan, but they grow wild in many warm subtropical to tropical areas in eastern and southern Asia, including China and Indonesia.

This fat-free, virtually zero-calorie food, which has been used as an ingredient in Japanese dishes for over 2,000 years, consists of 97% water and 3% glucomannan, a fiber in the form of a viscous substance. It also has some traces of protein, starch and minerals like calcium.

It's the glucomannan content that has the effect of eliminating a considerable percentage of the calories you eat. Glucomannan is an amazingly dense high-fiber substance that has the ability to expand to 200 times its size upon entering the digestive tract. It binds calories, carbohydrates and fats in fiber. Therefore, as these food particles pass through your digestive system, the body regards them as fiber, and flushes them out of your body, along with the toxins in the digestive tract. It's no wonder the Japanese call it a "broom for the stomach."

Scientific Evidence Proves that Glucomannan Enables Overweight or Obese People to Lose a Significant Amount of Weight

Several randomized placebo-controlled trials have studied the effects of glucomannan on weight loss. The largest of these studies involved 176 healthy but overweight subjects on a calorie-restricted diet, who were randomly assigned either a glucomannan supplement or a placebo. (https://pubmed.ncbi.nlm.nih.gov/15614200). The results after 5 weeks clearly proves that **glucomannan induced body weight reduction in healthy overweight subjects.** Weight loss was significantly greater among the study subjects who supplemented with glucomannan.

Several other studies corroborate these results. Glucomannan caused modest weight loss in overweight and obese individuals when regularly ingested before a meal.

In a study titled *Glucomannan and obesity: a critical review* (https://pubmed.ncbi.nlm.nih.gov/16320857), glucomannan was well-tolerated and resulted in **significant weight loss in overweight and obese individuals**.

In 14 studies investigating the effects of Glucomannan on body weight (https://pubmed.ncbi.nlm.nih.gov/18842808), glucomannan appears to beneficially affect body weight, as well as total cholesterol, LDL cholesterol, triglycerides, and FBG (fasting blood glucose).

An eight-week double blind trial titled *Effect of glucomannan on obese patients: a clinical study* (https://pubmed.ncbi.nlm.nih.gov/6096282), tested purified glucomannan fiber as a food supplement in 20 obese subjects. Glucomannan fiber (from konjac root) or placebo was given in 1-gram doses (two 500 mg capsules) with 8 oz water, 1 hour prior to each of three meals per day. Subjects were instructed not to change their eating or exercise patterns. Results showed a significant weight loss using glucomannan over an eight-week period. Serum cholesterol and low-density lipoprotein cholesterol were significantly reduced in the glucomannan treated group. No adverse reactions to glucomannan were reported.

When you take 2 to 4 capsules of glucomannan (totaling 2000mg or more) with a full glass of water 30 minutes before your "self-indulgent meal of the day," it not only supports healthy weight loss but also expands in your stomach and prevents you from overeating. Note: The number of capsules you take depends on the strength of the glucomannan product you're using, bearing in mind that you must consume 2000mg of glucomannan or more.

The "Self-Indulgent Meal of the Day"

Eat any food you want—with just <u>one tiny twist</u> (hara hachi bu) that accelerates weight loss.

One of the main reasons most weight loss programs fail to deliver long-term results is because people on a diet feel *deprived* of the food they want to eat. When faced with deprivation, which is an **unnatural** state to be in—especially in our land of plenty—most people quit and return to their old eating habits with a vengeance.

What's even worse is when people cheat on their diets—and feel **guilty** about it. Psychologists have discovered that if you are racked with guilt while eating (or after eating) something you're not allowed to eat, you have a higher likelihood of gaining more weight than if you enjoyed the food without feeling guilty. The emotional stress caused by the feeling of guilt makes you pile on the pounds more than the calories you'd have consumed from eating the forbidden food.

Study findings published in the online edition of the journal *Appetite*, show that the way we *perceive* tasty treats like chocolate cake is just as important as the calorie count when it comes to expanding waistlines. So if you're going to indulge in food anyway, make sure you enjoy every crumb (instead of feeling guilty) in order to minimize weight gain.

Most weight loss programs now allow for one "cheat day" a week. The reasoning falls along these lines: When you are allowed a cheat day on your diet once a week, you are able to look forward to being rewarded on "cheat day"—and you then don't feel so deprived by your restrictive diet. Whoever invented "cheat day" thought that having one day a week to eat as you please would make you less likely to give in to temptation to binge during diet days, and help you stick to your diet on a long-term basis.

Unfortunately, things rarely turn out that way, as evidenced by the majority of people who abandon their diets, even if they're allowed one cheat day a week.

In this regard, the Pound-a-Day Rapid Weight Loss program may be the polar opposite of the standard weight loss program because it allows you to have one self-indulgent meal each day. Every day is "cheat day"—and you'll never have feelings of deprivation or guilt—ever. For lunch, you can eat anything you want (within reason)—but on one condition: **You can eat only until you're 80% full**.

How likely are you to stick to a weight loss program if you get to eat what you want in at least one meal a day? Might you be inclined to stick to the program forever? Once you see the Pound-a-Day Rapid Weight Loss Program in its entirety, I think you'll say, "Absolutely!"

Eating until you are only 80% full is a cultural habit practiced on the island of Okinawa, Japan, a place where more people are living longer and healthier than anywhere else on earth.

Scientists are convinced that this practice of not eating until completely full is one reason for the astonishing longevity of Okinawans. In Okinawa, elders call this way of eating *hara hachi bu*, which loosely translates to "eat until you are 8 parts full [out of 10]." It's a practice cited by researchers as one of the reasons that more people in Okinawa live past 100 than anywhere else.

"If you think of a single mechanism that would explain why caloric restriction seems to extend not only life span but health span, it would be reduction of free radicals, because less food is being metabolized for energy." This, according to Bradley Willcox, a Mayo Clinic-trained internist and a geriatrics fellow in Harvard University's Division on Aging.

Observations of the life-extending benefits of calorie restriction go far beyond Okinawa. An enormous body of research confirms the longevity benefits of eating less. According to an article in *Science Daily*:

> In studies going back to the 1930s, mice and many other species subsisting on a severely calorie-restricted diet have consistently outlived their well-fed peers by as much as 40%.

When you have one daily meal wherein you eat anything you want (within reason)—but only until you're 80% full, you're training your body to curb your own appetite. Within 21 days, it becomes a habit, and then a way of life. In due time, you'll notice your food consumption will be healthier than it used to be. When faced with an all-you-can-eat buffet, you're less likely to binge on unhealthy food, and less likely to fill your plate to overflowing—or go back for second helpings— just because you can. It makes you more mindful of what you're putting into your body, and tempers any overactive appetite that you might have. In time, you'll find that you begin to make healthier food choices.

Once you begin to lose weight rapidly on this weight loss program, you'll realize that the following popular saying is true:

> **Nothing tastes as good as being thin <u>feels</u>.**

The foods you love will change as you become more conscious of what the quantity and quality of food does to your body and your energy level. You may find that you'll spontaneously choose healthier alternatives to the "unhealthy" foods you used to love. To help you on your way to conscious eating, I've presented recipes in Chapter Five for healthy versions of popular foods like pizza, burgers, fries, Mac 'n Cheese, hotdogs, chips, and meatloaf.

Why You Must Chew Your Food Slowly—and Chew Your Food More

It has long been known that when you eat your food too fast, you end up consuming more calories than you would if you ate at a slower pace. Here's why: Our body has a way of telling us when we need to eat to ensure survival, and also when we are full and need to stop eating.

The feeling of hunger comes from the hypothalamus, which plays a role in the amount of food our body consumes. The feeling of fullness (satiety) is often associated with how the stomach feels, but it actually has more to do with the hypothalamus.

As the stomach begins to fill up with food or water, stretch receptors in the stomach are activated, which send a signal to the brain. Hormonal signals (such as cholecystokinin and leptin) are released as partially digested food enters the small intestine—and in response to food consumed during a meal. These hormones amplify the signals to the brain, enhancing the feeling of fullness. When you eat too quickly, you are not giving the satiety signal from the hormones enough time to register in the brain.

Since the feeling of satiety comes from the brain, not from the stomach, the amount of food in your stomach is only one of the factors involved in the satiety process. It takes approximately 20 minutes time for the body to tell the brain that it has had enough food; and only when the body has sent this signal to the brain can the brain activate the satiety response (which originates in the hypothalamus) that makes us stop eating. Therefore, if you wolf down your food in less than 20 minutes, you're overshooting your actual point of satiety, and you'd have eaten too much before the brain told your body to stop eating.

Therefore, one of the best ways to make sure you eat only until you're 80% full is to chew your food slowly, thereby allowing the satiety signal to kick in before you've eaten too much.

In a recent study, the results of which were published in *The Journal of Clinical Endocrinology & Metabolism*, scientists reported that when a group of subjects was given an identical serving of ice cream on different occasions, they released more hormones that made them feel full when they ate it in 30 minutes instead of five minutes. The scientists took blood samples and measured insulin and gut hormones before, during and after eating. They found that two hormones that signal feelings of satiety (or fullness) showed a more pronounced response in those who ate slowly, which led to eating less.

Another study published in *The Journal of the American Dietetic Association* in 2008 revealed similar findings. In that study, subjects reported greater satiety and consumed roughly 10 percent fewer calories when they ate at a slow pace compared with times when they gobbled down their food. In yet another study published in *The British Medical Journal* involving 3,000 participants, those who reported eating fast (and eating until full) had **triple the risk of being overweight** compared with others.

The second way to ensure that you eat only until you're 80% full is by chewing your food more.

New research conducted at Iowa State University proves that when you chew your food slowly—chewing plays an essential role in the digestion process, influencing the absorption of nutrients and bringing about feelings of satiety or fullness.

The researchers studied 20 Iowa State students who were given a metronome and instructed to chew in time with the ticking of the metronome. Half of the participants chewed 15 times and the other half 40 times. Researchers took blood samples to study plasma glucose levels and hormones, and monitored the subjects' appetite. They found that the subjects who chewed more consumed less food.

> "When people chewed the pizza 40 times before swallowing, there was a reduction in hunger, preoccupation with food and a desire to eat," the researchers reported. "There was an increase in CCK, which is a hormone related to fullness and satiety. And there was a reduction in ghrelin, another hormone that stimulates the brain to increase appetite."

The researchers also found plasma glucose and insulin levels were higher among the subjects who chewed the pizza 40 times. **They surmised that the increased mastication breaks down the food more thoroughly in the mouth, and this facilitates nutrient absorption.** This has the effect of getting more glucose and carbohydrates into the bloodstream, which requires a larger insulin response to maintain plasma glucose levels.

The third way to ensure that you eat only until you're 80% full is to follow this rule of thumb for portion control: Put food on your plate equivalent to approximately half (50%) of what you normally eat in a normal meal. Eat your food slowly and chew your food thoroughly, and by the time you've finished the food on your plate, you will most likely feel full, and you won't want to eat more food.

Remember: If you've already had the 2 to 4 capsules of the glucomannan (totaling 2000mg) with a glass of water, plus you've had approximately 50% of the food you normally eat in a meal, that would be roughly equivalent to eating only until you're 80% full.

Pu-Erh Tea

*Scientifically proven to **shrink fat cells**, increase metabolism, help shed water weight, and prevent the body from turning the food you eat into fat*

Pu-erh is a broadleaf tea varietal that comes from Yunnan province in southwestern China, where there is a town called Pu'er, near the borders of Vietnam, Laos, and Myanmar (formerly called Burma). The tea is made from a miraculously versatile strain of *camellia sinensis* called Dayeh, which are ancient trees with mature leaves that are known to be between 500 and 1000 years old.

The history of pu-erh tea (pronounced *poo-air*) can be traced back about two centuries to the Han dynasty. To this day, this tea remains quite popular in China and some other parts of Asia. It is one of the very few exotic teas that improves with age, much like fine wine. Some varieties of pu-erh that are 30 years old, for example, command prices in excess of a $1,000 per pound. The famed Peninsula Hotel in Hong Kong serves pu-erh tea at a premium price of $18.00 for a small pot.

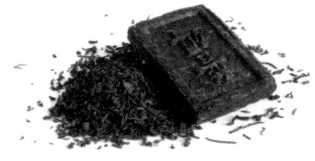

In more recent years, pu-erh tea has been scientifically proven to **shrink fat cells**, increase metabolism, help shed water weight, and prevent the body from turning the food you eat into fat.

It is pu-erh tea's ability to suppress fatty acid synthesis that helps prevent weight gain and obesity. Scientific studies found that consumption of pu-erh tea leaves significantly suppressed the expression of fatty acid synthase (FAS) in the livers of rats. It also suppressed weight gain, as well as levels of triacylglycerol and total cholesterol.[1][2]

These findings were corroborated by a study conducted in the Institute of Biochemistry and Molecular Biology, College of Medicine National Taiwan University, Taipei, wherein researchers studied the effects of feeding four kinds of tea to young rats. The tea varieties included pu-erh,

---

[1] Chiang, Chun-Te; Weng, Meng-Shih; Lin-Shiau, Shoei-Yn; Kuo, Kuan-Li; Tsai, Yao-Jen; Lin, Jen-Kun (2005). "Pu-erh tea supplementation suppresses fatty acid synthase expression in the rat liver through down-regulating Akt and JNK signalings as demonstrated in human hepatoma HepG2 cells." Oncology research 16 (3): 119–28. PMID 16925113.

[2] Lin, Jen-Kun; Shoei-Yn Lin-Shiau (September 28, 2005). "Mechanisms of hypolipidemic and anti-obesity effects of tea and tea polyphenols". Molecular Nutrition & Food Research (Weinheim: WILEY-VCH Verlag GmbH & Co. KGaA) 50 (2): 211–217. doi:10.1002/mnfr.200500138. PMID 16404708.

oolong, black and green tea. They found that the tea that exhibited the highest efficacy in suppressing the test rats' body-weight gains compared with those of the control rats was pu-erh tea. Weight loss occurred in the test rats despite the fact that there were no significant differences in total food intake among the test and control groups of rats. Furthermore, specific mechanisms through which chemicals in pu-erh tea inhibit the biosynthesis of cholesterol in the laboratory have been suggested. [3]

A randomized, double-blind, placebo-controlled study gave 59 overweight or mildly obese subjects either three grams of pu-erh extract per day or a placebo for 20 weeks. The researchers found that the tea extract was "associated with **statistically significant weight loss** when compared to placebo."

Fat loss was observed in the arms, legs and the hip/belly region of subjects. Mild reductions in cholesterol were also observed in the subjects who took the pu-erh extract.

Additional Scientific Evidence that Pu-Erh Tea Reduces Body Fat

In 1986, Japanese researchers conducted a study involving the effects of pu-erh tea and conventional green tea on lipid (fat) metabolism in rats whose diet contained 1% cholesterol by weight. Although neither the green tea nor the pu-erh tea had any significant effect on the rats' body weight, the pu-erh group had a **significant reduction of adipose tissue (body fat)**, both in absolute terms and as a percentage of body weight. Green tea had no effect on body fat reduction. Furthermore, the plasma levels of triglycerides (fat molecules) were reduced in the pu-erh group but not in the green tea group.[4]

In a 20-week randomized placebo-controlled study conducted at NIS Labs in 2016, (https://www.ncbi.nlm.nih.gov/pmc/articles/PM-C4818050), researchers found about a **3% reduction in total body fat** in the control group when compared to the placebo group, which experienced no change. There were no other dietary restrictions imposed on the subjects.

---

[3] Lu, Chi-Hua; Hwang, Lucy Sun (1 November 2008). "Polyphenol contents of Pu-Erh teas and their abilities to inhibit cholesterol biosynthesis in Hep G2 cell line". Food Chemistry 111 (1): 67–71. doi:10.1016/j.foodchem.2008.03.043.

[4] Sano M, Takenaka Y, Kojima R, Saito SI, Tomita I, Katou M, Shibuya S. Effects of Pu-erh tea on lipid metabolism in rats. Chem Pharm Bull 1986;34:221-8.

Traditional Uses of Pu-Erh Tea

Many people drink pu-erh tea because there is also ample evidence that:

- Pu-erh reduces bad cholesterol and lowers triglycerides. In one study conducted on laboratory animals, pu-erh tea was the only kind of tea which could actually **raise the level of good cholesterol** (HDL) and **lower the level of bad cholesterol** (LDL). American chef and restaurateur Alice Waters, who is regarded as the "mother of California cuisine," stated in a *Financial Times* interview that pu-erh tea has lowered her cholesterol 100 points. "It was extreme," she said. "You have to try some."

The microbial aging of pu-erh tea has been shown to result in the production of lovastatin, a natural statin. Statins are a class of drugs that act to reduce levels of fats, including triglycerides and cholesterol, in the blood. One study found that the longer the pu-erh tea was aged, the higher the level of statin produced.

- Pu-erh may help to reduce blood sugar
- Pu-erh reduces arteriosclerosis, reduces plaque in the heart, and helps to prevent strokes.
- Pu-erh improves circulation.
- Pu-erh is a source of antioxidants which help fight cancer and promote cell health
- Pu-erh has anti-inflammatory properties, including the amino acid GABA, which may help to alleviate arthritis, asthma and arteriosclerosis. The chemical theophylline, which is naturally occurring in tea leaves, is a key component in some asthma medications.

Pu-erh tea has been used to control weight for more than 1,700 years. It was only recently that it piqued the interest of the scientific community; and research studies, such as those described above, have proven its weight loss merit. In February, 2012, Dr. Mehmet Oz, cardiothoracic surgeon, *New York Times* bestselling author and television personality, who is also called "America's Doctor," recommended on his *Dr. Oz* TV show that people drink a couple cups of pu-erh tea a day to aid in weight loss.

The pu-erh tea one consumes on the Pound-a-Day Rapid Weight Loss program should ideally be derived from **organic** pu-erh leaves that have been aged in the dark, humid caves of the Yunnan province for at least 5 years. After the leaves are dried and rolled, they go through microbial fermentation, which means that microbes work on the tea leaves in a fashion similar to the fermentation of wine or cheese. This causes the leaves to darken, grow rich in flavor, and deliver tea that has a sweet, woodsy aroma and mild earthy finish. **If it's made any other way, it's not authentic pu-erh**.

Post-fermentation by aging also breaks down the caffeine levels in pu-erh, meaning that the caffeine content naturally diminishes, the older it gets. This indicates that a very old pu-erh might have trace amounts of caffeine by the time it is consumed, in comparison to a younger pu-erh.

The actual caffeine content present in a cup of organic pu-erh tea varies depending on how long the tea is steeped. The longer the steep time, the more caffeine the tea will contain. Caffeine content will lessen each time the tea bag is re-steeped or used again. For weight loss purposes, the ideal steep time for organic pu-erh tea is 5 minutes.

Note: Some black teas, which are neither from the Yunnan province nor aged the way pu-erh leaves are traditionally aged, are passed off as pu-erh tea by unscrupulous tea vendors. Beware of such purveyors of "fake" pu-erh tea, which doesn't deliver the benefits of authentic pu-erh.

Organic Chia Seeds

*The best overall weight control and appetite control
for losing one pound a day*

There's a humble seed from a Mexican plant, which has recently emerged as a superfood that delivers miraculous health value. This seed called chia, comes from the *Salvia Hispanica* plant, which has been known for its health benefits since the days of the ancient Aztecs.

Chia seeds were a main component of the Aztec and Mayan diets because of their complete nutritional profile and astonishing energy benefits. Aztec warriors could reportedly survive for 24 hours of combat on just 1 tablespoon of chia. Traditional healers in present-day Mexico continue to use chia in the treatment of a wide range of health conditions.

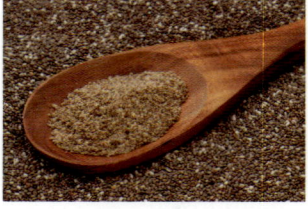

Chia seeds are a uniquely beneficial seed classified as a *food* by the Food and Drug Administration (FDA), and regarded by many as the "**world's healthiest whole raw food.**" Their health benefits are backed by over 30 years of scientific and agricultural research.

In the last 15 years, the miraculous health benefits of chia seeds have been hailed and recognized by doctors, health practitioners, nutritionists, scientists, herbalists, and health enthusiasts. One look at chia seeds' nutritional profile, and the reason becomes apparent.

Chia seeds have the highest combination of omega-3 fatty acids, proteins, antioxidants, fiber, and phytonutrients of any source on the planet. They are also high in fiber and contain ...

- Twice as much potassium as bananas
- **6X more calcium than milk**
- More antioxidants than blueberries
- 2X more fiber than bran flakes
- 15X more magnesium than broccoli
- 4X more selenium than flaxseed
- **6X more protein than kidney beans**
- 9X more phosphorus than whole milk
- **8X more Omega-3s than wild salmon**
- **3X more iron than spinach**

Bob Arnot, M.D., the *New York Times* bestselling author of fourteen books on nutrition and health, and a medical correspondent for *NBC Nightly News*, *Dateline NBC*, the *Today* show, *CBS Evening News*, *60 Minutes*, and *CBS This Morning*, wrote the book, *The Aztec Diet: Chia Power: The Super Food That Gets You Skinny and Keeps You Healthy*. He has become an evangelist of the weight-reducing power and immense health value of chia seeds. He calls these seeds "the best overall weight control and appetite control" that he's ever found in a product.

Drink This Instead of Eating That!

For weight loss purposes, Dr. Arnot simply puts organic chia seeds in plain drinking water. Since micro-milled chia seeds absorb 12 times their own weight in water, they expand in your stomach, making you feel full. And **they provide much more nutritional value than the average meal**. That's why chia seeds mixed in water are **often used as a meal**

replacement. Dr. Arnot easily lost one pound a day using organic chia seeds mixed in water or almond milk.

As for nutrient value, Dr. Arnot said, "I could eat ten bowls of Brussels sprouts, cauliflower, spinach, or broccoli—or four scoops of chia. What a no brainer! What an incredibly easy way to pack in nutrients and lose weight without consuming massive amounts of vegetables!"

Because chia seeds have no taste that might turn off people with picky palates, practically anyone can use these seeds to lose weight. The standard Pound-a-Day Rapid Weight Loss program calls for replacing the evening meal with a chia drink consisting of one scoop (or 2 tablespoons – 13 grams) of organic chia seeds in water. But you can also replace the self-indulgent lunch meal with the chia seed drink to accelerate weight loss.

He also believes chia seeds may be one way to "beat the terrible epidemic of obesity" that we have in the U.S. and across the Western world.

Chia Seeds Might Make You Lose Too Much Weight!

Dr. Arnot created his own nutritional challenge using organic chia seeds. He had weighed as much as 225 pounds when his wife was pregnant with their first son. He was able to go down to 208 pounds by trying all types of diets. But when he got to 208 pounds, he was stuck. He couldn't lose any more weight no matter how hard he tried, no matter how much he starved himself, or how much he worked out. He would sometimes go down to 203 pounds, but before long, he would be back to 208 pounds again. He tried all the diets he could find, but he just couldn't lose those stubborn 15 pounds to achieve his goal weight. So he tried to stop eating in the late afternoon every day because he knew he could lose weight by skipping dinner. But whenever he skipped dinner, he would suffer brain-drain from low blood sugar, and the hunger pangs would send him to the kitchen, raiding the fridge for whatever food he could find.

When he discovered organic chia seeds, it changed everything. He would have a scoop at 3:00 PM, and nothing for dinner. And surprisingly, he had no hunger pangs, no loss of brain energy, and no shaky feeling of low blood sugar. Since then, he has lost one pound a day whenever he wanted to. In fact, he had to hold himself back because he was **losing too much weight too quickly**. He eased up on the chia seeds in order to lose weight more slowly. Before long, his weight went down to his goal weight of 188 pounds. He was not only healthy and lean, but he had so much energy that he was able to work long hours and do intense workouts on cross-country skis, downhill racing skis, bikes, and paddleboards.

Not All Chia Seeds Are Created Equal

The best chia seeds to use when you're on the Pound-a-Day Rapid Weight Loss program are those that are capable of delivering all the weight loss and health benefits summarized in this book. Ideally, the chia seeds should have the following attributes:

1. The chia seeds should be derived from an extraordinary strain of *Salvia Hispanica* that has been shown to have **far higher nutritional values** than other strains of chia.
2. The chia seeds should be **certified organic** by the U.S. Department of Agriculture (USDA), are non-GMO (Genetically Modified Organism), and free of gluten, pesticides and trans-fats. Clearly, organic chia seeds that are also non-GMO and gluten-free provide superior health benefits.

Organic chia seeds also have a broad spectrum of important health benefits. They have been shown to slow down the aging process of your body ... control Type II diabetes ... prevent heart disease ... relieve arthritis ... inhibit cancer tumors ... normalize blood pressure ... stop hair loss ... overcome depression ... reduce chronic pain ... eliminate acid reflux ... banish constipation ... get rid of fatigue and low energy ... or help heal practically any health condition.

There are amazing stories online of people who have done these things—and more—successfully through organic chia seeds.

It is a documented fact that food cravings occur due to a deficiency in vitamins and minerals in the body. Because organic chia seeds are so nutrient-dense, they help balance the nutrient quotient in your body, thereby enabling you to curb cravings.

Another way organic chia seeds help you shed excess weight is through their rich supply of omega-3 fatty acids. It's a proven fact that consuming this healthy fat makes you lose body fat. A study conducted at the University of South Australia proved that subjects who took omega-3 fatty acids lost weight, as reported in *Natural News*.

The study involved 75 participants, who were diagnosed as being either overweight or obese, and split into four groups. After three weeks, three of the groups did not show much change, but the group that was given the omega-3 fatty acids had an average weight loss of about 4.5 pounds and a decrease in overall body fat percentage. This was so, even though no other changes in eating habits were made.

To use chia seeds as part of the Pound-a-Day Rapid Weight Loss program, put a scoop (approximately 2 tablespoons) of organic chia seeds in 16 ounces (2 cups) of water; stir, and set aside for about 3 minutes, allowing the mixture to thicken slightly. Drink this beverage—instead of having an evening meal.

Optional: In order to boost the nutritional content of the chia seed evening drink further, I recommend adding a scoop of nutrient-dense superfood powder. (See Recommended Websites and Resources for suggested superfood supplements.)

Should you weigh-in every day?

Ideally, you should weigh yourself at the beginning of your Pound-a-Day Rapid Weight Loss journey; that is, on the morning of Day 1. This will provide you with a good baseline weight to track how well you've progressed by the end of each week or month.

Important: Always weigh yourself first thing in the morning BEFORE you've had any food or drink, and AFTER you've emptied your bladder and had your daily bowel movement.

That's because there are many factors that can cause your weight to *appear* to have gone up an extra pound or two, which is what I call *fake weight*. These factors include fecal matter (which could weigh up to 2 pounds when unevacuated from your large intestines), constipation, hormonal fluctuations, water retention, menstruation, or even flatulence.

Always weigh yourself naked, or if you can't weigh yourself naked, wear the same clothes for consistency.

During your first week on the Pound-a-Day Rapid Weight Loss program, weigh yourself only at the end of that first week. Thereafter, you can weigh yourself every day.

Weighing yourself daily can be useful because you can learn a lot about how different factors cause your weight to fluctuate day to day, such as what you eat and drink (and what time), exercise, using the toilet, or if you're a woman, your menstrual cycle. You might also find daily weigh-ins motivating because you'll get to see the pounds fall away everyday as long as you stay on track.

Nonetheless, daily weight fluctuations are sometimes inevitable. If these fluctuations are stressful to you, or trigger anxiety and excessive preoccupation with your weight, weighing-in at the end of each week would be more appropriate for you.

"Pound-a-Day is the only weight loss program that has ever worked for me. I don't even feel like I'm on a diet because I can eat anything I want, and yet I lost 19 pounds in just over 5 weeks, and I continue to lose weight like clockwork every week. I also lost 5 inches off my waist, 6 inches off my hips, and I went down 2 pant sizes in 3 weeks! All in all, I've lost a total of 17 inches from my upper body in just a few weeks, and now I stand tall again because I've regained the confidence I lost so long ago!" -- A. Mercer, Schaumburg, Illinois

Chapter Three

Fast Track Your Way to Even Faster Weight Loss

Lose a dress or pant size in one week

The Pound-a-Day Rapid Weight Loss™ program enables you to lose weight even though you have one "self-indulgent meal of the day" wherein you can eat anything you want—as long as you eat until you're only 80% full, take 2 capsules of glucomannan with a full glass of water before the meal, and 2 cups of pu-erh tea after. If, in addition to that, you're also taking at least one green smoothie and one chia seed drink a day, it's almost impossible not to lose weight.

However, if you really want to accelerate your weight loss to one pound a day or more, follow the three simple guidelines below. Following these guidelines will speed up your weight loss while also supporting vibrant health.

1. Double the number of times you take the chia seed drink. If you're following the standard Pound-a-Day Rapid Weight Loss program, you can choose to have a chia seed drink instead of your self-indulgent meal of the day (lunch).

Many of those who've had significant weight loss on this program were busy people who lost a tremendous amount of weight ... *accidentally.* Some of these people had jobs that kept them tied to their desks eight hours a day or out in the field, and they rarely had time to even have lunch. Therefore, in order to tide themselves over, they put 2 tablespoons of organic chia seeds in a glass of water, and drank it—while telling themselves they'd grab lunch later when they had a free moment. More often than not, they forgot about having lunch altogether because the chia drink made them feel as though they had a full meal. And they found that replacing the noontime meal with the chia drink, in addition to replacing the evening meal also with a chia drink, made them lose more than two pounds a day—and they rarely got hungry.

The difference between having a chia drink and a traditional meal replacement drink from processed powder is this: The chia drink contains a powerhouse of nutrients far superior to the nutritional value one gets from an average meal. As mentioned in Chapter Two, Dr. Bob Arnot equated four scoops of chia seeds to ten bowls of Brussels sprouts, cauliflower, spinach, or broccoli. And Dr. Arnot found himself **losing too**

much weight too quickly on chia seeds alone. Wouldn't everyone wish they had that problem?

Additionally, the human body recognizes chia seeds as food because they <u>are</u> food, which many health advocates regard as the world's healthiest raw food. In contrast, most commercial meal replacement powders are processed products that are enriched with synthetic (and isolated) vitamins, minerals and nutrients, artificial ingredients and added sugar that the human body does not recognize as food. Therefore, such nutrients are often excreted because the body is unable to absorb or utilize them.

2. Double the number of daily servings of glucomannan. The standard Pound-a-Day Rapid Weight Loss plan recommends taking 2 to 4 capsules (totaling 2000mg) of glucomannan with a full glass of water 30 minutes before the noontime "self-indulgent meal of the day." To accelerate weight loss, take 2 capsules of glucomannan also before you consume the green smoothie in the morning.

3. Choose healthier versions of the foods you love. When you do eat your self-indulgent meal of the day, if you crave comfort foods like burgers, fries, pizza, Mac 'n Cheese, hotdogs, or meatloaf, have the healthy (and less calorific) versions of these foods instead. See healthy recipes for all your favorite foods in the recipe section of this book.

<u>*Optional*</u>: *If you feel inclined to skip your self-indulgent meal of the day, replace it with a second green smoothie.*

"I never get hungry after the Pound-a-Day chia seed drink I have for dinner every night. When I wake up each morning, I feel light as a feather and full of energy, not sluggish the way I used to be. I lost 15 pounds in 30 days, and was able to slim down just in time for my daughter's wedding! I also experienced tremendous health benefits. My blood sugar level normalized -- previously averaging 150-170, and now between 98 and 110. Under my doctor's direction, I've stopped taking insulin shots -- didn't need them anymore. My doctor has also cut my diabetic medication (Metformin) by half -- from two 1000mg tablets down to two 500mg tablets. Plus, my blood pressure also normalized -- previously, my BP upon waking up used to be 148/86 -- and now, it's at 120/80 or below. This has allowed me to stop taking some of my meds and lower the dosage of others." -- Katerina D., New Rochelle, New York

4. Engage in strength training. The Pound-a-Day Rapid Weight Loss program alone will enable you to lose weight successfully—even if it's not combined with exercise. However, if you <u>also</u> do strength training while you're on the program, you will **greatly increase the speed of your weight loss effort**. In fact, when you do strength training (in the form of high-intensity interval training), you might even **double the effectiveness** of the Pound-a-Day Rapid Weight Loss program. Here's why:

When you engage in high-intensity interval training (also called HIIT), you build muscle. The mere existence of muscle in your body burns more calories from the food you eat—and also burns more body fat around the clock, even while you sleep.

How much time does it take to do high-intensity interval training? It takes **as little as 20 seconds** per muscle group per week. When you engage one muscle group with a 20-second high-intensity contraction, your body gets the signal that it needs that muscle, so it will then hold on to it instead of letting that muscle tissue waste away.

Why is this important? When you lose muscle tissue as a result of any weight loss program, you sabotage your own weight loss efforts because your body becomes less metabolically efficient, and starts to burn food at a slower rate. On the other hand, short bursts of high-intensity interval training send the message to your body that it needs to hold on to your muscle mass.

Chapter 8 of this book features the *20-Second Workout*, a vastly improved version of High-Intensity Interval Training that includes not only strength training, but also super-cardio exercises, flexibility, balance and stability training. Only one of the exercises in the 20-Second Workout is isolated (i.e., targets one muscle); the rest are highly effective **compound** exercises (i.e., target multiple muscle groups at once), which make for more time-efficient workouts that burn body fat and build lean muscles.

High-intensity interval training will make you gain muscle, but women need not worry that it will make the body bulk up or develop bulging muscles (thereby making them look bigger and fatter). If anything, HIIT will give firmness, tone and definition to your body—which are what give the body an awesome shape. FACT: Fat takes up to 5 times as much space as muscle in your body. So as long as you're losing fat on the Pound-a-Day Rapid Weight Loss program, you will experience weight loss—even as you gain muscle, which takes up less space in your body.

<u>Note</u>: *When you engage in high-intensity interval training, your weighing scale may not be the best way to measure the success of your weight loss*

efforts. Because muscle weighs more than fat, you may actually gain weight if you engage in high-intensity interval training. But the additional muscle will accelerate fat loss, and you'll see the difference in the number of inches (not pounds) that you lose.

Here are additional tips for accelerating weight loss:

WEIGHT LOSS TIP #1:
Eat nutrient-dense super foods.

It is a well-known fact that when you're well-nourished, you don't get hungry. When you're eating nutritious food—even in small quantities that don't quite fill your stomach to capacity—you feel satiated and not hungry. However, if you indulge in foods with empty calories—even in quantities that fill your stomach beyond its normal capacity—you might feel satisfied for an hour or two; but before long, you'll be craving your next fix. No amount of empty food will do because your body is looking for sustenance that nourishes it. And eating a huge amount of junk food —or taking a multivitamin pill—cannot fill that need.

The ideal strategy for satisfying your body's need for sustenance without having to stuff your body with a huge amount of food is to consume nutrient-dense superfoods, such as blueberries, spinach, pistachio nuts, red bell peppers, beans, oats, pumpkin, spirulina, chlorella, moringa, wheatgrass, cacao, maca, acai, and camu-camu.

Because these superfoods are not usually included in meal recipes, the next best thing is to use a superfood powder blend that contains some or all of these superfoods, and add a scoop to your green smoothie or to your chia seed drink. Some of the best superfood powder blends are listed in the *Recommended Websites and Resources* section of this book.

WEIGHT LOSS TIP #2:
Avoid consuming ultra-processed foods (UPF).

A food isn't necessarily bad for you just because it's processed in some way. Minimally processed foods, for instance, are those with added vitamins or minerals, or maybe a little bit of sugar or harmless additive.

Ultra-processed foods, (UPF), on the other hand (also called highly processed foods), are foods that have been altered to include a patchwork of ingredients (such as fats, starches, sugars, salts, preservatives, additives and hydrogenated oils extracted from other foods).

These ingredients are meant to enhance the taste and flavor of the food, make the food more shelf-stable (i.e., last longer in your pantry before expiring), and engineered by food scientists to be extremely addictive. It's how they keep consumers buying and eating these foods and making them staple products that households stock at home all the time.

A study published online (*Nutrients*, June 30, 2020) titled *Ultra-Processed Foods and Health Outcomes: A Narrative Review*, revealed the following conclusion:

A high dietary intake of ultra-processed foods is associated with a range of adverse health outcomes, diseases, disorders and conditions, including the following:

- Overweight, obesity and cardio-metabolic disorders
- Cancer (breast, ovarian, colorectal, all cancers)
- Cardiovascular disease
- Coronary heart disease
- Cerebrovascular disease
- Type 2 diabetes
- Gastrointestinal disorders
- Depression
- Asthma
- Death (a **31% higher risk of all-cause mortality**)

Another recent study showed that consumption of ultra-processed foods are directly responsible for approximately 11 million deaths worldwide every single year.

Ultra-processed foods that you <u>must</u> avoid -- not just to support your weight loss goals but also to protect yourself from the aforementioned list of health hazards -- are the following:

> Pre-packaged soups, sauces, frozen pizza, ready-to-eat meals, hot dogs, sausages, french fries, sodas, store-bought cookies, cakes, candies, doughnuts, ice cream, sweetened breakfast cereals, flavored potato chips, white bread, fried chicken, flavored candy bar with long ingredient list, frozen, blended coffee drink, mashed potato flakes, energy drink, flavored granola bars with added sugar and preservatives, artificially flavored cheese crackers, and ultra-processed meats, such as ham, bacon, salami, hotdogs, beef jerky and corned beef.

It's best to consume minimally processed food, or better still, homemade food that you make yourself using healthy ingredients. Chapter 5 features homemade (i.e., healthier) alternatives to ultra-processed foods like burgers, fries, Mac 'n Cheese, meatloaf, pizza, hotdogs and spaghetti.

WEIGHT LOSS TIP #3:
Avoid eating foods that contain Monosodium Glutamate (MSG)

MSG is in 80% of all flavored foods that you get at a restaurant, at the supermarket, and at most retail establishments. Most people don't realize that MSG causes an effect that is counterproductive to weight loss: It makes you want to eat more. Furthermore, MSG is an excitotoxin containing brain-damaging poisons, which seriously threaten your health. But more importantly, MSG excites the part of your brain which is in charge of the fat program, and due to that excitation, your body activates the fat program, causing the body to accumulate fat. Scientists know this because when they conduct studies on obesity, they need obese laboratory mice; and, the way to fatten up a mouse is by feeding it MSG—and the result is a study subject called "MSG obesity-induced mice."

So avoid MSG at all costs, if weight maintenance is important to you. On food labels, marketers usually disguise the MSG content by calling MSG a host of other names, including Hydrolyzed Vegetable Protein, Hydrolyzed Protein, Hydrolyzed Plant Protein, Plant Protein Extract, Sodium Caseinate, Calcium Caseinate, Yeast Extract, Textured Protein, Autolyzed Yeast, Hydrolyzed Oat Flour, Malt extract, Malt flavoring, Bouillon, Broth, Stock, Flavoring, Natural Flavoring, Natural Beef or Chicken Flavoring, Seasoning, Carrageenan, Soy Protein Concentrate, Soy Protein Isolate, and Soy Protein Concentrate.

WEIGHT LOSS TIP #4:
Avoid Fat-Free Foods

In an ostensibly valiant effort to help curb the trend of the general population from getting fatter than it already was, food companies started to make a great many food products fat-free. The word "fat-free" on a food label means it's loaded with sugar (to gain back the taste of the food which was diminished when the fat was removed). When sugar is ingested, it turns to fat in the body. That's because it first elevates the sugar levels, causing the pancreas to secrete insulin in order to reduce the blood sugar. And insulin is a fat-producing hormone. Fat is really good for you if it's the right kind of fat.

Misinformed nutritionists and so-called fitness experts always seem to proclaim that as far as weight loss is concerned, all fats will make you fat, and should be avoided at all costs. Actually, the contrary is true: **Not eating fats will make you fat.** When you limit your fat intake, you are training your body to start storing fat—and this could *ironically* lead to excessive body fat.

Healthy fats include food items that have essential fatty acids like Omega-3 (chia seeds, flax seeds, green leafy vegetables, salmon, Atlantic halibut, sardines, albacore tuna, Atlantic mackerel, lake trout, shellfish) and Omega-6 (sunflower seeds, sesame seeds, most nuts, animal meats and some fish).

Bad fats that you must avoid include saturated fats (butter, lard, the fat on steak), trans fats, which are vegetable oils that are hydrogenated (margarine, shortening and partially hydrogenated vegetable oil). Even oils that sound "healthy," such as soybean oil, canola oil and corn oil, need to be avoided because these are not healthy for you to consume in large quantities on a long-term basis.

WEIGHT LOSS TIP #5:
Avoid consuming artificial sweeteners and products that contain artificial sweeteners (such as aspartame).

Most people who want to lose weight reach for the artificial sweetener aspartame (NutraSweet) instead of sugar to sweeten their tea or coffee because they erroneously think it is a healthier choice. They think so because aspartame has zero calories, and therefore, won't cause them to gain weight. This is untrue. Artificial sweeteners such as aspartame not only interfere with the body's ability to count calories, but they also promote sugar cravings, are addictive, and lead to weight gain.

Aspartame is present not only in artificial sweeteners, but is also an ingredient in more than 6000 popular food products (including diet colas), most of which are marketed as "sugar-free" or "diet" products. Long-term aspartame consumption not only sabotages your weight loss efforts, but also causes brain imbalances, oxidative stress, and even brain tumors, according to a study published in *Drug and Chemical Toxicology*. Aspartame reactions also include stomach pains, nausea, insomnia, sluggishness, headaches/migraines, panic attacks, impaired vision, and depression.

Artificial sweeteners appear in product labels not only as aspartame, but also saccharin, sucralose, acesulfame potassium (acesulfame-K), and neotame.

It's also advisable to avoid the "natural sugar substitutes" like Truvia and Purevia because they're highly processed. A natural sweetener that's worth considering is Stevia, a sweet, zero-calorie substance that comes from the stevia shrub.

WEIGHT LOSS TIP #6:
Avoid consuming commercial fruit juices and products that contain high fructose corn syrup (HFCS).

In the 1970s Japanese scientists developed the technology to separate fructose (fruit sugar) from corn, thus creating a sweetener called high-fructose corn syrup (HFCS) that was so much cheaper than sugar. HFCS is now present in thousands of food products (including salad dressings, pasta sauces, frozen pizza), soft drinks, and commercial fruit juices. Recent findings have revealed that consuming HFCS is far worse than consuming sugar. A high-fructose diet can cause you to build new fat cells around your heart, liver, and digestive organs in just 10 weeks, and triggers the early stages of diabetes and heart disease, according to a 2009 study from the University of California, Davis. By comparison, a high-glucose diet did not have the same effects.

Excessive consumption of HFCS-laden food and drinks leads to increased belly fat, insulin resistance, metabolic damage, as well as a long list of chronic diseases.

WEIGHT LOSS TIP #7:
Don't eat meals while you're watching TV or while working.

When you do this form of "unconscious" eating, you'll invariably feed yourself more than you need to (which could cause weight gain)—and you won't enjoy the food you're eating.

WEIGHT LOSS TIP #8:
Drink plenty of water!

Thirst is often confused with hunger. When you think you're hungry, reach for a glass of water first. It will most likely eliminate psychological hunger, and help reduce the food/calories you consume.

How to determine how much water you should drink daily:

Drinking 8 glasses of water a day is a myth. Every person is different, and optimum water consumption should be a factor of your body weight—if your goal is to lose weight.

Here's the water consumption formula for weight loss: Take half your body weight, convert that to ounces—and that's the amount of water you should drink.

Example 1: If you're a woman who weighs 112 pounds:

Divide 112 by 2 = 56

56 ozs divided by 8 (since there are 8 ozs per glass of water) = 7 glasses of water per day

Example 2: If you're a man who weighs 160 pounds:

Divide 160 by 2 = 80

80 ozs divided by 8 (since there are 8 ozs per glass of water) = 10 glasses of water per day

If this seems like a lot of water to you, it certainly is. But if you do nothing else but drink your recommended amount of water, you will accelerate your weight loss results by two to four additional pounds lost per month—or more. The only downside to it is that it will cause you to urinate often. But remember that every single time you urinate, you rid your body of ugly fat, unwanted waste and toxins.

MISCELLANEOUS WEIGHT LOSS TIPS:

⇒ Don't eat after 7:00 PM (to allow food to be digested before going to bed)

⇒ Don't eat when stressed, sad or angry (to avoid emotional food cravings)

⇒ Portion Control Trick: Eat from a plate, never from a bag or boxes. Buy small size plates in colors that decrease your appetite (e.g., brown, grey, black).

⇒ Have a shopping list before going to the supermarket or grocery store. A list helps to avoid buying and eating unnecessary, unhealthy or fattening food. And remember: Don't go to the grocery store when hungry.

⇒ Remove all junk food from your home and work place.

⇒ Don't just monitor the pounds you lose on the Pound-a-Day Rapid Weight Loss program, but also check the inches you lose. Ideally, record your measurements (waist, hips, thighs) before you start on the program. Measure every week to see your progress.

⇒ Get a diet buddy to go on the Pound-a-Day Rapid Weight Loss with you. You'll keep each other motivated, and keep yourself accountable to each other.

⇒ To accelerate weight loss further, and achieve a more chiseled body with definition, do the 20-Second Workout, a modified version of High-Intensity Interval Training (HIIT) 1 to 3 times a week. The entire 20-Second Workout is a perfect adjunct to the Pound-a-Day Rapid Weight Loss program, and is featured in its entirety in Chapter 8.

Chapter Four

Customize the Pound-a-Day Rapid Weight Loss Program™ for Your Specific Lifestyle

Why you can "cheat" any day of the week and still lose weight

Unlike other weight loss programs that require you to stick to a strict plan or diet, the Pound-a-Day Rapid Weight Loss program allows you countless ways to customize the plan to suit your specific lifestyle and preferences—and still achieve your weight loss goals.

Outlined below are just three customized plans that abide by the principles of Pound-a-Day Rapid Weight Loss program, followed by guidelines for creating a custom plan just for you:

———•———

Customized Plan A: This is suitable for people who must eat dinner, and who don't think they'll be satisfied with just having the chia seed drink as a dinner replacement. This customized plan is ideal for busy parents who need to synchronize their meal times with those of their families; individuals who workout and need additional protein; and individuals who stay up late at night.

1) Take a 16-oz glass of water upon waking up in the morning. *(Optional: Add the juice of half a lemon and a dash of cayenne pepper to the water to give your metabolism a jump start.)*

2) Mid-morning: Have a 16-oz green smoothie consisting of 60% fruits and 40% green leafy vegetables. *(Optional: If you're going to be out for a few hours and want the feeling of fullness to last longer, include 1 tbsp of organic chia seeds in your green smoothie.)*

3) Thirty minutes before lunch, take 2 to 4 capsules (or a total of 2000mg) of glucomannan (from Konjac Root) with a full glass of water.

4) For lunch, you can eat leftovers from the day before or have any food you want (within reason), as long as you **eat only until you're 80% full**.

5) Take 2 cups of organic pu-erh tea immediately after lunch.

6) Mid-Afternoon or Post-Workout Snack: Have an 8 oz whey protein shake with water or almond milk. *Tip: Always choose a whey protein that is non-GMO, contains no artificial sweeteners or sugar. If you're really hungry, put a scoop (2 Tablespoons) of organic chia seeds in your shake.*

7) Pre-dinner: Thirty minutes before dinner, take either 2 to 4 capsules (2000mg) of glucomannan with a full glass of water or a chia seed drink (2 tablespoons of organic chia seeds in 16 ozs of water).

8) Dinner: The glucomannan or chia seed drink will help you eat a significantly reduced amount of food for dinner. Eat as healthy a meal as possible (see recipes in Chapter Five for ideas), and follow the guideline of eating only until you're 80% full. Make sure you're done eating dinner no later than 7:00 PM.

9) Pu-Erh Tea: After dinner, have one cup of pu-erh tea to prevent the food you ate from turning into fat. *Note: Only one cup is advised (as compared to two cups after lunch) because pu-erh contains caffeine and may interfere with your sleep, if you consume too much of it at night.*

10) After-dinner snack (optional): If you stay up late at night and have a craving for sweets, have a sugar-free dark chocolate bar followed by a tall glass of water. (See *Recommended Websites and Resources* for information on Choco Perfection, the chocolate bar voted the No. 1 Best-Tasting Sugar-Free Chocolate.) If you have a craving for something other than sweets, have a 14- gram bag of SkinnyPop Non-GMO, Gluten-Free Popcorn, a small handful of raw almonds or unsalted mixed fancy nuts, followed by a tall glass of water.

Customized Plan B: This is suitable for people who are always on the road and don't have time to prepare a green smoothie; and individuals who often eat their meals in their car, in between appointments or meetings, or on the go.

1) Take a 16-oz glass of water upon waking up in the morning. *(Optional: Add the juice of half a lemon and a dash of cayenne pepper to the water to give your metabolism as jump start.)*

2) Mid-morning: Have a chia seed drink (2 tablespoons of organic chia seeds in 16 ozs of water).

3) Thirty minutes before lunch, take 2 to 4 capsules (or 2000mg) of glucomannan (from Konjac Root) with a full glass of water.

4) For lunch, you can grab a fast food lunch on the road—but make sure you choose healthy menu items, such as gluten-free, non-GMO and low-calorie options, if available, and **eat only until you're 80% full**.

5) Take two cups of organic pu-erh tea immediately after lunch.

6) Mid-Afternoon Snack (optional): Have an 8 oz whey protein shake with water or almond milk. *Tip: Always choose a whey protein that is non-GMO, contains no artificial sweeteners or sugar. If you're really hungry, put a scoop (2 Tablespoons) of organic chia seeds in your shake.*

7) Ideally, you should have a chia seed drink (16-oz glass of water with 2 tablespoons of organic chia seeds) instead of dinner. But if you must have dinner with clients, co-workers, friends, or family members, take 2 to 4 capsules (or 2000mg) of glucomannan with a full glass of water or a chia seed drink 30 minutes before dinner. For dinner, choose healthy menu options and follow the guideline of eating only until you're 80% full. It may not always be possible to finish dining before 7:00 PM, but when you have the choice, dine as early in the evening as possible and avoid late-night dining.

8) Pu-Erh Tea: After dinner, have one cup of organic pu-erh tea to prevent the food you ate from turning into fat. <u>Note</u>: *Only one cup is advised (as compared to two cups after lunch) because pu-erh contains caffeine and may interfere with your sleep, if you consume too much of it at night.*

9) After-dinner snack (optional): If you stay up late at night and have a craving for sweets, have a sugar-free dark chocolate bar followed by a tall glass of water. (See *Recommended Websites and Resources* for information on Choco Perfection, the chocolate bar voted the No. 1 Best-Tasting Sugar-Free Chocolate.) If you have a craving for something other than sweets, have a serving of SkinnyPop non-GMO, gluten-free popcorn), a small handful of raw almonds or unsalted mixed fancy nuts, followed by a tall glass of water.

Customized Plan C: This is suitable for people who have more active professions like service providers, those involved in construction, contractors and subcontractors, and those who work long days, and have to grab meals wherever they happen to be.

1) Take a 16-oz glass of water upon waking up in the morning. *(Optional: Add the juice of half a lemon and a dash of cayenne pepper to the water to give your metabolism as jump start.)*

2) Mid-morning: Have a 16-oz green smoothie consisting of 60% fruits and 40% green leafy vegetables. *(Optional: If you're going to be out for a few hours and want the feeling of fullness to last longer, put 1 tbsp of organic chia seeds in your green smoothie.)*

3) Thirty minutes before lunch, take 2 to 4 capsules (or 2000mg) of glucomannan (from Konjac Root) with a full glass of water.

4) For lunch, you can eat a bagged lunch that you prepared (see easy-to-prepare meals in Chapter Five, which you can eat cold). Or you can eat leftovers from the previous day. If you grab a fast food lunch on the road, make sure you choose healthy menu items, such as gluten-free, non-GMO and low-calorie options, if available, and **eat only until you're 80% full**.

5) Take 2 cups of oganic pu-erh tea immediately after lunch.

6) Mid-Afternoon Snack (optional): If you crave sweets, have a sugar-free dark chocolate bar followed by a tall glass of water. (See *Recommended Websites and Resources* for information on Choco Perfection, the chocolate bar voted the No. 1 Best-Tasting Sugar-Free Chocolate.) If you crave something salty, have a serving of SkinnyPop non-GMO, gluten-free popcorn, or 10 lightly salted roasted almonds, followed by a tall glass of water.

7) Ideally, you should have a chia seed drink (16-oz glass of water with 2 tablespoons of organic chia seeds instead of dinner. But if you must have dinner with clients, co-workers, friends, or family members, take 2 to 4 capsules (or 2000mg) of glucomannan with a full glass of water or a chia seed drink 30 minutes before dinner. For dinner, choose healthy menu options and follow the guideline of eating only until you're 80% full. It may not always be possible to finish dining before 7:00 PM, but when you have the choice, dine as early in the evening as possible and avoid late-night dining.

8) Pu-Erh Tea: After dinner, have one cup of oprganic pu-erh tea to prevent the food you ate from turning into fat. <u>Note</u>: *Only one cup is advised (as compared to 2 cups after lunch) because pu-erh contains caffeine and may interfere with your sleep, if you consume too much of it at night.*

———•———

As you can see from the three customized plans above, it's just a matter of mixing up the components of the Pound-a-Day Rapid Weight Loss program to suit your lifestyle. If you're the kind of person who likes to have three square meals a day, for example, you can customize the plan and allow yourself to get accustomed to it gradually, as follows:

Day 1: Pick one of your meals—any meal (breakfast, lunch or dinner)—and replace them with one of these Pound-a-Day Rapid Weight Loss "meals":

⇒ A green smoothie consisting of 60% fruits and 40% green leafy vegetables (preferably organic); or

⇒ A "Self-Indulgent Meal of the Day" wherein you eat anything you want (within reason), but **eat only until you're 80% full**. This meal should be preceded by 2 to 4 capsules (2000mg) of glucomannan taken with a full glass of water 30 minutes prior to the meal; and followed by two cups of organic pu-erh tea immediately after the meal; or

⇒ A chia seed drink consisting of 2 tablespoons of organic chia seeds in a 16-oz glass of water.

For your 2 other meals of the day, have what you usually have.

Day 2 through 7: Repeat what you did on day 1.

Day 8 through 14 (Week 2): Pick two of your meals (breakfast, lunch or dinner)—and replace them with one of these Pound-a-Day Rapid Weight Loss "meals":

⇒ A green smoothie consisting of 60% fruits and 40% green leafy vegetables (preferably organic); or

⇒ A "Self-Indulgent Meal of the Day" wherein you eat anything you want (within reason), but **eat only until you're 80% full**. This meal should be preceded by 2 to 4 capsules (2000mg) of glucomannan taken with a full glass of water 30 minutes prior to the meal; and followed by 2 cups of organic pu-erh tea immediately after the meal; or

⇒ A chia seed drink consisting of 2 tablespoons of organic chia seeds in a 16-oz glass of water.

For your third meal of the day, have what you usually have.

Day 15 through 21 (Week 3): Do exactly what you did in Week 2, but with 2 additional conditions: 1) One of your "meals" should consist of only the chia seed drink (2 tablespoons of organic chia seeds in a 16-oz glass of water); and, 2) If you're having dinner, make sure you're done with dinner before 7:00 PM.

Day 22 through 28 (Week 4) and beyond: Do exactly what you did in Week 3.

When you gradually ease into the Pound-a-Day Rapid Weight Loss program as described above, and allow yourself the freedom to mix and match your choice of "meals," you'll find your own comfort zone, and you'll also discover for yourself which components are enabling you to lose the most weight so you can adjust your program accordingly.

Chapter Five

28 Days of Nutritionally Balanced Recipes

Delicious, kitchen-tested recipes with weekly shopping lists

This chapter features 28 days of nutritionally balanced meal recipes that are not only delicious, but will also support your weight loss goals—especially if you use one of these 28 recipes as your "Self- Indulgent Meal of the Day."

The recipes include homemade (and healthier!) alternatives to store-bought—and usually ultra-processed—foods like burgers, fries, Mac 'n Cheese, meatloaf, pizza, hotdogs and spaghetti.

Almost all of the recipes can be prepared in 30 minutes or less (except the meatloaf, which takes 45 minutes). Each recipe yields 2 servings.

If you want just one serving, divide the ingredients by two, or better still, prepare the meal for two, eat half of it today, and save the other serving for tomorrow. If you want more servings for a family of 4, for example, just double the ingredients indicated in the recipe.

> # WEEK 1:
> ## Recipes for Meat Eaters and Non-Vegetarians

Week 1 – Monday

Smoked Salmon and Cheese on Sweet Potato Crust

Servings: 2

Cook time: 35 minutes

<u>Ingredients</u>:

<u>Toppings</u>:

3 ounces cold smoked salmon, cut into thin strips

¼ cup sliced red onion

1 sliced green pepper

½ cup crumbled goat cheese

Zest of 1 lemon

<u>For the crust</u>:

1 medium sweet potato

1 egg

1 cup rolled oats

½ cup almond flour

2 tablespoons flaxseeds

1 tablespoon olive oil

1 tablespoon baking powder

Salt and pepper to taste

<u>Directions</u>:

Preheat the oven at 375° F

In a blender mix together the potato, rolled oats, almond flour, egg, baking powder, flax seeds, salt and pepper.

Spread the olive oil evenly on a pizza tray. Place the mixture on the tray, and bake 25-30 minutes at 375° F

Remove the pizza from the oven, add the toppings (salmon, green pepper, red onion and goat cheese) and bake for 5 more minutes.

Healthy tip: Sweet potatoes have low glycemic index (which means they do not cause blood sugar to spike quickly). Foods that have a high glycemic index—like white potatoes or bread—have been associated with type 2 diabetes, cardiovascular diseases, obesity and certain cancers.

Week 1 – Tuesday

Grilled Turkey Burgers

Servings: 2

Cook time: 30-40 minutes

Ingredients:

    1 lb turkey, minced

    ⅓ cup quinoa

    1 egg

    2 tablespoons sweet chili

    1 clove garlic, minced

    ½ teaspoon fresh or dried parsley leaves

    2 large tomatoes

    ½ cup baby spinach

    Mustard, salt and pepper to taste

Directions:

Combine ⅔ cups water with quinoa in a saucepan and bring to a boil. Reduce the heat and simmer for about 15 minutes.

Combine turkey mince with cooked quinoa, egg, sweet chilly, garlic and parsley in a bowl and mix well. Add salt and pepper to taste.

Make 2 large patties out of this mixture and place them on the grill over medium high heat for 7-10 minutes, then flip to the other side and cook until done.

Cut the tomatoes in a half and use them instead of burger buns. Place the burger on a half, add mustard and baby spinach and place the other half on top.

Healthy tip: Turkey meat (especially if you choose breast turkey) is a healthier option because it has less fat and calories compared with traditional beef burgers. Grilled is also better than fried; plus, the turkey will cook faster.

Week 1 – Wednesday

Mashed Cauliflower with Baked Chicken Drumsticks

Servings: 2

Cook time: 35 minutes

Ingredients:

- 4 chicken drumsticks (skinless)
- 1 tablespoon olive oil
- 1 teaspoon coconut oil
- ½ tablespoon fresh rosemary
- 1 small head cauliflower chopped (about 4 cups)
- ½ cup plain yogurt
- Salt and pepper to taste

Directions:

Preheat the oven at 425° F

Rinse and pat dry drumsticks. Rub the drumsticks with one tablespoon of olive oil, salt, pepper and rosemary. Place the drumsticks on a baking sheet.

Bake for 15 minutes, rotate each drumstick and bake for another 10-15 minutes (or until done).

While the chicken is cooking in the oven, bring a pot of salted water to a boil.

Add the cauliflower and cook (until very tender) for about 7 minutes. Leave a few tablespoons of water, and drain the rest.

Using a blender mix the cauliflower with water, coconut oil and ½ cup of yogurt until smooth.

Add salt and pepper to taste.

Healthy tip: Mashed cauliflower is a great alternative to mashed potato—equally tasty, but with less calories and carbs. You can use coconut oil (that helps you lose weight) to replace the butter (that promotes weight gain) not only in this recipe, but anytime and with any other meals that include butter.

Week 1 – Thursday

Guilt-Free Baja Fish Tacos

Servings: 2

Cook time: 20 minutes

Ingredients:

- 2 frozen or fresh fish fillets 4 oz each (i.e. tilapia)
- 2 medium corn tortilla
- ½ cup red cabbage, shredded
- 1 tablespoon olive oil
- ½ red onion, sliced
- 1 clove garlic, diced
- 1 teaspoon chopped jalapeños
- A pinch of ground cumin
- Salt and pepper to taste

Directions:

Preheat the oven at 400° F.

Place the fish on a baking dish covered with olive oil.

Bake fish fillets in the oven 15-20 minutes (or until fish flakes easily with a fork). Remove from the oven.

(If you choose soft tortillas, you may want to place them in the oven for 5-10 minutes as well, while cooking the fish)

In a bowl combine the cabbage with onion, garlic, cumin, and jalapeños.

Cut the fillets into small strips, and place them on tortilla. Add cabbage mixture from the bowl on top.

Healthy tip: These guilt-free tacos provide a good balance of protein-carbohydrate-fats. If you adopted a gluten-free lifestyle, double check if the corn tortillas indeed don't have gluten added. Jalapeños (the capsinoids) help speed up the metabolism, curb your appetite and aid in the weight loss.

Week 1 – Friday

Chicken Schnitzel with Cabbage and Avocado Salad

Servings: 2

Cook time: 30 minutes

Ingredients:

- 2 medium, thin chicken cutlets
- 1 egg
- 2 tablespoons milk
- 2 tablespoons almond flour
- 1 + 1 tablespoons olive oil
- 1 tablespoon lime juice
- 1 cup shredded fresh cabbage
- 1 avocado, diced

Directions:

Preheat the oven at 400° F

In a bowl whisk together egg and milk.

Lightly coat the chicken cutlets in flour, shake the excess flour, then dip the cutlets in egg mixture. Sprinkle a dash of salt.

Place the chicken cutlets on an oven tray coated with one tablespoon olive oil. Bake for 30 minutes (or until chicken is tender). Remove from oven.

In a bowl mix shredded cabbage, avocado with one tablespoon of olive oil, lime, salt and pepper. Serve with the schnitzels.

Healthy tip: Oven-baked schnitzels taste as good as the fried ones, but are much healthier. Cabbage salad can be used with meals, or by itself, anytime you feel hungry, and it helps you lose weight. Red cabbage is even better for blood sugar control because it contains natural pigments called anthocyanins (that boost insulin production and lower sugar levels).

Week 1 – Saturday

Chicken Breast with Veggies

Servings: 2

Cook time: 20 minutes

Ingredients:

    1 + 1 tablespoons olive oil
    2 slices (6 ounce) breast chicken, skinless
    ½ tablespoon parsley, chopped
    ½ cup tomatoes, diced
    ½ cup kalamata olives, chopped, pitted
    ½ cup red bell peppers, diced
    1 teaspoon lemon juice
    2 soft tortillas
    Salt and pepper to taste

Directions:

Preheat the grill for medium heat and lightly oil grate.

Place the chicken on grill for 10 minutes, than flip it onto the other side for 10 more minutes or until done.

While cooking the chicken, in a bowl combine one tablespoon of olive oil, the olives, tomatoes and red pepper and lemon juice.

Remove chicken from heat, place each piece on a tortilla and add the vegetable mixture on top. Add salt and pepper to taste.

Healthy tip: You may crave that crispy, high-saturated-fat chicken skin. With this recipe you won't miss it, because kalamata olives and the olive oil are a great replacement.

Week 1 – Sunday

Baked Chicken Wings

Servings: 2

Cook time: 20 minutes

Ingredients:

    2 boneless, skinless chicken breast halves, cut into strips
    1 tablespoon olive oil
    ⅓ cup almond flour
    1 garlic clove, crushed
    1 cup milk
    2 cups baby spinach
    One tablespoon lemon juice
    Salt to taste
    For Home Buffalo sauce (see recipe on page 94)

Directions:

Preheat the oven at 400° F

Combine the milk with almond flour and crushed garlic in a bowl.

Dip the chicken strips into the batter, and place them on a baking tray (lightly coated with olive oil).

Place the tray in the oven, and cook for 15-20 minutes (or until crisp)

In the meantime, prepare the Buffalo sauce: (see recipe on page 94)

Remove the tray from the oven, place the chicken in a bowl and toss with the sauce.

Serve with baby spinach drizzled with lemon juice.

Healthy tip: This recipe is a healthier, low-fat alternative to traditional chicken wings. Homemade Buffalo sauce replaces the unhealthy version found in the stores, and it can be refrigerated and used for up to 1-2 weeks.

WEEK 1 SHOPPING LIST:

3 ounces cold smoked salmon

2 frozen fresh fillets (tilapia)

4 halves breast chicken

4 chicken drumsticks

2 thin chicken cutlets

1 lb turkey

One bag white onion (small)

One bag garlic (small)

One red onion

One green bell pepper

2 lemons

One lime

1 medium sweet potato

2 large tomatoes

One bag (bunch) baby spinach

One cauliflower

One small red cabbage

One small green cabbage

One avocado

Kalamata olives

Red bell peppers

Rolled oats

Almond flour

Flaxseeds

One bag quinoa

4 corn tortilla wraps

Eggs

Milk

1-2 small yogurts

Goat cheese

Sweet paprika

Chili

Cayenne pepper

One small bottle rice vinegar

Baking powder

Fresh parsley

One bunch fresh rosemary

Ground cumin

Jalapeños

> # WEEK 2:
> ## Recipes for Meat Eaters and Non-Vegetarians

Week 2 – Monday

Pizza with Pesto, Chicken and Tomato

Servings: 2

Cook time: 35 minutes

Ingredients:

- 2 medium corn tortilla wraps
- 1 teaspoon olive oil
- 1 chicken breast half
- ¼ cup pesto
- ½ cup tomatoes, diced
- 2 tablespoons tomato sauce
- 1 cup feta cheese crumbled
- Salt and pepper to taste

Directions:

Preheat the oven at 375° F

Cut the chicken breast into small strips and place in a sauce pan.

Add 1 cup of water and boil it over medium high heat. When done (in about 10 minutes), drain through a sieve into a bowl.

Place the tortilla wraps on an oven tray, lightly coated with olive oil. Coat the wrap with tomato sauce, and top with chicken strips, tomatoes, feta cheese and pesto. Add salt and pepper to taste.

Bake for 25 minutes. Remove from oven and serve.

> **Healthy tip:** Chicken breast can easily dry out when grilled or baked, thus boiling it is a great option. Tortilla wraps have less calories and carbs compared to the regular dough, and are also gluten-free.

Week 2 – Tuesday

Savory Amaranth and Tuna

Servings: 2

Cook time: 25 minutes

Ingredients:

- 1 can tuna fish (in water)
- ⅓ cup amaranth grain
- ½ cup leeks, sliced
- ¼ head broccoli
- 1 tablespoon olive oil
- Salt and pepper to taste

Directions:

Add ⅓ cup amaranth to 1 cup of boiling water over medium high heat. Cover the pan with a lid, reduce heat.

Add broccoli, leeks and pepper and let simmer until water is fully absorbed (15-20 minutes).

Remove from the heat, combine with olive oil, add tuna on top and serve.

Healthy tip: This recipe is a great alternative to a tuna sandwich. Amaranth contains three times more fiber than wheat, and is an excellent source of calcium and iron. The whole seeds can be popped like popcorn and used as a snack.

Week 2 – Wednesday

Turkey Meatballs with Bok Choy

Servings: 2 (8 meatballs)

Cook time: 25 minutes

Ingredients:

> ½ lb ground turkey
>
> ¼ cup onion, sliced
>
> clove garlic, minced
>
> 2 teaspoons parsley, finely chopped
>
> 2 teaspoons soy sauce, low sodium
>
> 1 egg, lightly beaten
>
> For bok choy:
>
> 2 heads baby bok choy, trimmed, leaves separated
>
> 2 teaspoon olive oil
>
> 1 teaspoon lemon juice
>
> Salt and pepper to taste

Directions:

Preheat the oven at 400° F

In a bowl mix the ground turkey with onion, garlic, parsley and egg. Add salt and pepper to taste (use little salt, because soy sauce will be added).

Form the balls by rolling 1 tablespoon of the mixture between your palms. Place them on an oven tray and cover them with soy sauce. Bake for 20 minutes (or until fully cooked).

Toss bok choy, oil and salt in another oven tray. Roast for 5-6 minutes. Remove from the oven, add lemon juice and pepper. Serve with turkey meatballs.

Healthy tip: This is a healthier alternative to Chinese food. Buy lean turkey and ask the butcher to grind it fresh—much better than buying ground turkey already in package (you never know what's inside!)

Week 2 – Thursday

Baked Tilapia and Veggie French Fries

Servings: 2

Cook time: 25 minutes

Ingredients:

    ½ lb tilapia fillets

    1 tablespoon parsley leaves

    ½ lemon, sliced

    1 tablespoon + 1 teaspoon olive oil

    For carrot chips:

    ½ lb carrots cut into French fry style sticks

Directions:

Preheat oven at 425° F

Rinse fish and pat dry. Place in a single layer on an oven tray lightly coated with olive oil. Add salt and pepper to taste.

Bake for 15-20 minutes (or until crisp tender). Remove from oven, add the lemon slices and parsley.

While the fish is cooking, place the carrot sticks in a baking pan, lightly coated with olive oil. Bake for 15 minutes, until they are crisp and tender. Add salt and pepper to taste and serve with the fish.

Healthy tip: This recipe is a great alternative to fish and chips. Carrots have less carbs and calories, but more healthy fiber compared to potatoes. Note that carrots have more sodium, thus you should add less salt.

Week 2 – Friday

"You-Won't-Miss-the-Meat" Vegetarian Meatloaf

Servings: 2

Cook time: 45 minutes

Ingredients:

- 1 red bell pepper, finely chopped
- 1 tomato, diced
- 1 lb Portobello mushrooms, chopped
- 2 tablespoons olive oil
- ⅓ cup onion, chopped
- 1 can (15 ounces) pinto beans, drained
- ⅓ cup walnuts, toasted, chopped
- 1 egg, beaten
- Salt, pepper and mustard to taste

Directions:

Preheat oven at 400° F

Heat a non-stick skillet over medium high heat. Add the oil, then the mushrooms; after 4-5 minutes add the peppers and tomato and sauté until tender.

Place the beans in a blender and mix until almost smooth. In a bowl, combine the beans, chopped walnuts with mushroom mixture, eggs, olive oil, salt and pepper.

Spoon mixture into an oven pan coated lightly with olive oil. Bake for 35-40. Remove from oven and serve with mustard.

Healthy tip: This is a healthier alternative to conventional meatloaf, packed with healthy fats, proteins and carbs.

Week 2 – Saturday

Frutti di Mare (Seafood) with Salad and Quinoa

Servings: 2

Cook time: 20 minutes

Ingredients:

- 1 cup marinated seafood (shrimps, calamari, baby octopus, etc)
- 2 cups baby spinach leaves
- ⅓ cup quinoa
- 1 tablespoon olive oil
- 1 medium tomato, diced
- ¼ cup onion, chopped
- 1 clove garlic
- 1 tablespoon olive oil
- Salt and pepper to taste

Directions:

Combine ⅔ cup water with quinoa in a saucepan and bring to a boil over high heat. Cover, reduce the heat and simmer for about 15 minutes. Stir in tomatoes, and cook for few more minutes.

In the meantime, sauté onions and garlic in a saucepan over medium heat, 1 tablespoon olive oil.

Remove quinoa from the heat. Add the sautéed onion and garlic. Add salt and pepper to taste. Serve with baby spinach salad and marinated seafood (after draining the liquid).

Healthy tip: Although this appears to be a light meal, it is well-balanced (calorie- and nutrient- wise) and heart-healthy. The seafood is packed with vitamins and minerals and omega-3 fatty acids. Although seafood contains cholesterol, it will not have a significant impact on your cholesterol levels as the high-saturated fats found in red meat and processed foods do.

Week 2 – Sunday

Silky Chickpea Hummus with Eggplant Chips

Servings: 2

Cook time: 25 minutes

Ingredients:

- 1 cup chickpeas, canned and drained
- 1 clove garlic, minced
- 1 + 1 tablespoons olive oil
- 2 tablespoons lemon juice
- ½ cup sour cream or Greek yogurt
- Salt and pepper to taste
- 6 thin slices eggplant
- 4 romaine lettuce leaves

Directions:

Preheat oven at 275° F

Place the eggplant circles on a baking tray lightly coated with olive oil. Add salt and pepper to taste.

Bake for 20-25 minutes.

While eggplants are cooking in the oven, blend the chickpeas with garlic, olive oil, lemon juice, sour cream and 1/3 cup water in a blender until almost smooth. You may want to let it sit for 10 minutes before serving with eggplant chips and salad.

WEEK 2 SHOPPING LIST:

- 1 chicken breast half
- One can tuna fish (in water)
- ½ lb ground turkey
- ½ lb tilapia filets
- One small jar marinated seafood
- 3 tomatoes
- Tomato sauce
- 1 bunch leeks
- One bunch broccoli
- One small bag onions
- One small bag garlic
- 2 heads baby bok choy
- One small bag carrots
- 1 lb Portobello mushrooms
- One red bell pepper
- One bag (bunch) baby spinach
- 2 lemons
- One eggplant
- One bag romaine lettuce (hearts)
- 1 can pinto beans
- One can chickpeas
- 2 medium corn tortilla wraps
- One box amaranth
- One box quinoa
- Feta cheese
- Eggs
- One small yogurt (or sour cream)
- One small bag walnuts
- Pesto
- One small bottle soy sauce (low-sodium) or Bragg Liquid Aminos (a natural soy sauce alternative)
- One bunch parsley leaves

WEEK 3: Vegetarian-Friendly Recipes

Week 3 – Monday

Spaghetti Squash with Mushroom, Tomato Sauce and Cheese
vegetarian-friendly, vegan-friendly

Servings: 2-4

Cook time: 25 minutes

Ingredients:

- 2- 2½ lb spaghetti squash
- ½ cup crumbled feta cheese
- 2 medium (one large), chopped Portobello mushroom(s)
- 1 teaspoon minced garlic
- ¼ cup chopped onion
- 1 cup chopped tomatoes
- 1 tablespoon olive oil
- ½ cup chopped fresh parsley

Directions:

Preheat the oven at 375° F

Using a large, thick knife, cut the squash in a half lengthwise and place the halved squash cut side down on a baking pan.

Bake for 25-30 minutes at 375° (if you wish "al dente" texture; cook for another 15 minutes if you prefer it tender, however it can get mushy.)

In the meantime, prepare the sauce: heat the olive oil in a non-stick skillet over medium high heat. Add the mushrooms; after 5 minutes stir in onion, garlic and tomatoes and cook for a few more minutes. Remove pan from the heat and stir in parsley.

When the squash is ready, remove it from the oven and scoop out the seeds. Take a fork and scrape the squash out into strands that will look just like spaghetti. Add the sauce and the feta cheese on top and serve it while still warm.

Healthy tip: 1 cup spaghetti squash (cooked) has 4-5 times less calories, 4 times less carbohydrates, and more nutrients (like vitamin A and potassium) compared to pasta (cooked), and is also rich in healthy fiber.

Week 3 – Tuesday

Eggplant Meatballs with Baked Carrots
vegetarian-friendly, vegan-friendly

Servings: 2

Cook time: 40 minutes

Ingredients:

- ½ medium size eggplant, washed, dried, peeled and diced
- 1 tablespoon onion, diced
- 1 clove garlic, minced
- ½ cup canned black beans, drained
- ½ teaspoon oregano mixed with parsley (fresh or dried)
- 1 teaspoon nutritional yeast
- 1 egg
- ½ cup tomato sauce
- 2 medium carrots, cut into wedges
- Salt and pepper to taste

Directions:

Preheat the oven at 375° F

In a cooking pan sauté the onion for 5 minutes, then add the garlic and eggplant. Cook for about 10-15 minutes (until the eggplant is soft). Allow to cool.

In a blender add the eggplant mixture, the black beans, egg, oregano and parsley, salt and pepper. Blend until smooth.

Using a tablespoon, roll the mixture into balls (about 8 balls). Place the balls on a tray in the oven and cook for about 20 minutes, flipping half way from one side to another.

While cooking the eggplant mixture, on another tray, place the carrots, add a pinch of salt and pepper. It will also take about 20 minutes to bake them (will not be completely soft, but rather a bit crunchy).

In a small pot, heat the tomato sauce. When close to the boiling temperature, remove it from the heat. Add the nutritional yeast.

When the balls are ready, remove them from the oven, and add the tomato sauce. Serve with baked carrots.

Healthy tip: You won't miss the meatballs and French fries if you try this much healthier meal. Make sure the diced eggplant pieces are completely dry to avoid a mushy texture.

Week 3 – Wednesday

Popcorn & Stuffed Pepper

vegetarian-friendly, vegan-friendly

Servings: 2

Cook time: 10 minutes

Ingredients:

> For stuffed pepper:
>
> 2 small red bell peppers
>
> 1 cup Ricotta cheese
>
> ½ medium tomato, diced
>
> ¼ leek, finely chopped
>
> ½ cup alfalfa spouts
>
> For popcorn:
>
> ½ cup popcorn kernels
>
> 3 tablespoons coconut oil
>
> You will also need one large pot and a large bowl

To prepare popcorn:

Heat the pot over medium-high heat. Drop a few kernels and cover pot. When those few kernels start to pop, add the rest of them. Place the lid back on the pot, and shake the pot occasionally back and forth. When the popping slows, wait a few more seconds and remove the pot from heat. Wait a few more seconds and transfer the popcorn into a large bowl.

In a small pot, heat the coconut oil, until it becomes liquid. Drizzle the coconut, and sprinkle with salt and nutritional yeast.

To prepare stuffed peppers:

Cut each one in half, remove the seeds. In a bowl, combine ricotta cheese with tomato, leek, salt and pepper. Stuff the peppers with this mixture and add alfalfa sprouts on top.

Healthy tip: This quick and easy technique for preparing popcorn is a better alternative to microwaving popcorn, which "nukes" the food and depletes it of nutrients. Coconut oil is a tasty and healthier alternative to butter.

Week 3 – Thursday

Portobello Mushroom Veggie Burgers
vegetarian-friendly, vegan-friendly

Servings: 4 burgers

Cook time: 40 minutes

Ingredients:

- 2 + 1 teaspoons olive oil
- 1 egg
- ½ chopped onion
- ¼ minced garlic
- 2 medium sliced Portobello mushrooms
- 1 cup frozen or fresh mixed peas and carrots
- 1 tablespoon minced fresh parsley
- One 19 oz (540 ml) red kidney beans, rinsed and drained
- 1 cup shredded red cabbage
- ½ bag of bag tortilla chips
- Dijon Mustard, salt and pepper to taste

Directions:

Preheat the oven at 375° F

Heat 2 teaspoons olive oil in a non-stick skillet over medium high heat. Add the mushrooms; after five minutes stir in onion and garlic and cook for a few more minutes. Remove pan from the heat and stir in parsley.

Puree the kidney beans in a blender until smooth. Add the bean mixture to the mushrooms in the pan. Add the egg, peas and carrots as well as salt and pepper and combine. Cook for 10 minutes, stirring occasionally.

Remove the pan from heat and let the mixture cool down. Form the mixture into 4 patties. Place patties on a tray coated with 1 teaspoon of olive oil. Bake for 20 minutes and serve warm, on baked tortilla chips, topped with mustard and shredded red cabbage.

Healthy tip: This recipe makes delicious burgers that taste just like regular ones (because of the mushrooms and beans), but with less calories and fat. To avoid bloating or excessive gas associated with beans: before cooking them simply place them in a pot, add some water and a few slices of ginger and bring to a boil. Now they are ready to be used to prepare your meal.

Week 3 – Friday

Vegetarian Hotdogs
vegetarian-friendly, vegan-friendly
(vegan if excluding yogurt & cheese)

Servings: 2

Cook time: 30 minutes

Ingredients:

- 2 large carrots, peeled, ends trimmed
- 1 clove garlic, minced
- ⅓ cup soy sauce, low sodium
- 1 teaspoon Italian herbs
- ½ teaspoon brown sugar
- Salt and pepper to taste
- 2 corn (tortilla) wraps
- ½ cup sauerkraut
- ¼ cup onion, sliced
- 2 pickles, sliced
- 2 tablespoons Greek yogurt
- 1 teaspoon nutritional yeast or ⅓ tablespoon crumbled goat cheese

Directions:

Preheat the oven at 375° F

In a pan, place the carrots, add some water and bring to a boil. Cook for 7-10 minutes. Remove from heat.

Place the carrots in an oven tray; add soy sauce, sugar, garlic and Italian herbs. Bake at 375° for about 15-20 minutes, flipping halfway from one side to another.

Remove from the oven. Place the carrot dog on a tortilla, add sauerkraut, pickles, onions. Mix together the yogurt with nutritional yeast (or cheese) and add on top. Roll the tortilla into a wrap.

Healthy tip: The mixture of yogurt and nutritional yeast (or goat cheese) is a tasty, low-calorie, low-fat alternative to traditional mayonnaise, but with less calories and fat.

Week 3 – Saturday

Risotto

vegetarian-friendly

Servings: 2

Cook time: 25 minutes

Ingredients:

- 2 tablespoons olive oil
- ½ onion, chopped
- 1 garlic clove, minced
- 1 cup brown rice
- 3 Portobello mushrooms, diced
- 1 tablespoon parsley leaves, minced
- ½ crumbled feta cheese
- Salt and pepper to taste

Directions:

Bring 1 cup water and salt to rapid boil in a pan. Stir the rice into the water, reduce the heat to a simmer. Cover the pan to a lid and cook for 15-20, stirring occasionally. Remove from heat.

While cooking the brown rice, you can prepare the mushrooms. Heat the olive oil in a non-stick skillet over medium high heat. Add the mushrooms and after 5 minutes stir in the onion, garlic and cook for few more minutes. Remove pan from heat. Add salt and pepper to taste.

Add this mixture on top of the rice and stir in parsley and feta cheese.

> **Healthy tip:** Brown rice has less carbs, less calories and far more fiber than white rice. White rice is brown rice whose outer layer (the bran) has been removed. Brown rice helps you lose weight faster than white rice, and also ideal for diabetics.

Week 3 – Sunday

Polenta and Leeks

vegetarian-friendly, vegan-friendly

Servings: 2

Cook time: 35 minutes

Ingredients:

> ½ cup corn meal (polenta)
> 2 tablespoons crumbled feta cheese
> 1 egg
> 1 cup milk
> 1 + 1 tablespoons olive oil
> 2 leeks, sliced
> ½ cup tomato juice Salt to taste

Directions:

Combine water, milk and salt in a pan, and bring to a boil over high heat. Reduce the heat and slowly stir in the cornmeal. Use a wooden spoon and stir often for 15 minutes.

In a small bowl beat one egg. Add the egg and one tablespoon olive oil to the cornmeal, stir and cook for another 10 minutes, until the mixture is thick. Remove from heat; add the feta cheese on top.

Heat one tablespoon olive oil in a non-stick skillet over medium high heat. Add the leeks, cook for 5 minutes, then add the tomato sauce and cook for another few more minutes. Serve with polenta.

> **Healthy tip:** This is a great meal to have before or after a workout. Additionally, the corn (in the cornmeal) is superior to other grains in terms of carbs and calories; is easy to digest; and provides protein and fiber.

WEEK 3 SHOPPING LIST:

One spaghetti squash (2½ lb)

One can black beans

One can kidney beans

3 tomatoes

Tomato sauce

Tomato juice

One bag carrots

One eggplant

2 red bell peppers

7 Portobello mushrooms

One bunch leeks

One small box alfalfa sprouts

Fresh (or frozen) mixed carrots and peas

One small red cabbage

One bottle soy sauce (low-sodium) or Bragg Liquid Aminos (a natural soy sauce alternative)

Pickles (small jar)

Sauerkraut (small jar)

Brown sugar

Tortilla wraps

One bag corn tortilla chips

One box popcorn kernels

One bag brown rice

Corn meal (small box)

One bag nutritional yeast

One box feta cheese

One small box Ricotta cheese

Eggs

One small yogurt

Milk

One small bag garlic

One bag onions

One bunch fresh parsley

One bunch oregano

Italian herbs

Olive oil

Coconut oil (small jar)

Salt

Pepper

WEEK 4:
Vegetarian-Friendly Recipes

Week 4 – Monday

Quinoa Mac 'n Cheese
vegetarian-friendly

Servings: 2

Cook time: 20 minutes

Ingredients:

> ½ cup quinoa
> 1 tablespoon olive oil
> 1 medium tomato, diced
> ½ cup baby spinach
> ¼ cup onion, chopped
> 1 clove garlic
> ½ cup crumbled feta cheese
> 2 tablespoons nutritional yeast
> Salt and pepper to taste

Directions:

Combine 1 cup water with quinoa in a saucepan and bring to a boil over high heat. Cover, reduce heat and simmer for about 15 minutes. Stir in baby spinach, tomatoes, one tablespoon olive oil and cook for few more minutes.

In the meantime, sauté onions and garlic in a saucepan over medium heat, using 1 tablespoon olive oil.

Remove quinoa from the heat, Add the sautéed onion and garlic, as well as the nutritional yeast and mix well. Add salt and pepper to taste as well as the crumbled feta cheese.

Healthy tip: This recipe is not only a healthier, but also a tastier alternative to traditional Mac 'n Cheese. Quinoa is high in protein and fiber; and you will feel full and more energetic when quinoa is added to your meals.

Week 4 – Tuesday

Baked Omelette with Kale Chips

vegetarian-friendly

Servings: 2

Cook time: 30 minutes

Ingredients:

- 2 eggs (or 4 egg whites)
- ½ cup red bell pepper, cut in thin strips
- ½ cup green olives, sliced
- ½ cup goat cheese, crumbled
- ½ bunch kale (stems removed)
- 1 + 1 tablespoons olive oil
- Salt and pepper to taste

Directions:

Preheat the oven at 400° F

To prepare the omelette: Beat the eggs in a bowl, add the red pepper and the olives.

Pour the mixture into a baking pan lightly coated with olive oil. Bake for about 25 minutes, or until done. Sprinkle with goat cheese.

Wash kale and dry it very well (between paper towels to avoid getting soft and mushy). Tear the leaves in pieces (similar with small potato chips) and place them on a baking sheet in a single layer.

Spread the oil on the leaves with your fingers. Place in the oven and roast for 8-10 minutes (until crispy).

Healthy tip: Kale chips are a great low-carb, low-fat alternative to potato chips. Replacing two eggs with 4 egg whites will reduce unnecessary fats, while increasing your protein intake.

Week 4 – Wednesday

Veggie Hotdogs
vegetarian-friendly

Servings: 2

Cook time: 20 minutes

Ingredients:

    2 vegetarian hot dogs

    1 avocado, mashed

    ½ cup cucumber, diced

    ½ cup tomatoes, diced

    1 small carrot, shredded

    2 small zucchini, cut lengthwise in half, ends trimmed

    ½ cup crumbled feta cheese

    1 tablespoon olive oil

    Salt and pepper to taste

Directions:

Preheat the oven at 400° F

Place zucchini halves, skin side down on a baking sheet. Drizzle with oil, salt and pepper. Bake for 15-20 minutes.

Hot dogs can also be heated, by placing them in a baking pan, in the oven, for 10 minutes.

Remove from the oven, and scoop each half a bit, so the hot dog and the veggies will fit in. Use zucchini exactly like a hot dog bun, by placing the veggie hot dog, cucumber, tomatoes, shredded carrots and feta cheese in between 2 halves. Used mashed avocado instead of mayonnaise.

> **Healthy tip:** Choose gluten-free or wheat-free veggie hot dogs (read the labels). A gluten-free diet has been associated with reduced adipose (fat) tissue, inflammation and insulin resistance. See: http://www.ncbi.nlm.nih.gov/pubmed/23253599. Also read the section in this chapter titled *"Why Gluten-Free?"*

Week 4 – Thursday

Vegetarian Chili

vegetarian-friendly

Servings: 2

Cook time: 15 minutes

Ingredients:

- 1 teaspoon olive oil
- ½ cup onion, chopped
- 1 garlic clove
- ½ tablespoon chili powder
- ½ cup tomatoes, diced
- 2 tablespoons tomato paste
- 2 cans (15 ounce) mixed beans
- ½ cup feta cheese, crumbled
- 2 cups baby spinach
- ½ medium size bag corn chips, baked

Directions:

Heat oil in a pan over medium-high heat. Add onion and garlic and sauté for 3-5 minutes. Add the chili powder, tomatoes, beans and ½ cup water and stir to combine. Combine tomato paste with 2 tablespoons of water and add to the mixture. Bring to a boil and cook for 5-10 minutes.

Remove from heat, add cheese and serve with corn chips.

> **Healthy tip:** Add chili powder as much as you like, but not in quantities that will upset your stomach. It speeds your body's metabolism and thus aids weight loss.

Week 4 – Friday

Vegetarian Buffalo Wings
vegetarian-friendly

Servings: 2

Cook time: 25 minutes

Ingredients:

- 1 small cauliflower florets
- 1 + 1 tablespoons olive oil
- ⅓ cup almond flour
- 1 garlic clove, crushed
- 1 cup milk
- ½ cup feta cheese crumbled
- 1 tablespoon lime juice
- 1 (15 ounce) can black beans
- For Homemade Buffalo Sauce recipe, see page 94

Directions:

Preheat the oven at 420° F

Combine the milk with almond flour and crushed garlic in a bowl. Dip the cauliflower florets into batter and place them on a baking tray (lightly coated with olive oil). Place tray in the oven, and cook for 20 minutes (or more if you prefer the florets soft).

Place the mixture in a blender and blend until smooth.

Remove the tray from the oven, place the cauliflower in a bowl, add the cheese and toss the florets with the sauce.

In a bowl combine the black beans with lime juice, olive oil, salt and pepper. Serve with the cauliflower chicken wings.

> **Healthy tip:** This recipe is a much healthier alternative to chicken wings, with fewer calories and fat.

Week 4 – Saturday

Roasted Brussels Sprouts with Pecans
ced*vegetarian-friendly*

Servings: 2

Cook time: 15 minutes

Ingredients:

- 1 lb Brussels sprouts, trimmed, halved
- ½ cup pecans, roasted, chopped
- 1 tablespoon olive oil
- ½ clove garlic, minced
- 1 tablespoon lime juice
- 1 cup yogurt, plain
- 1 teaspoon nutritional yeast
- Salt and pepper to taste

Directions:

Preheat the oven at 375° F

On a baking tray toss the Brussels sprouts with pecans, oil, garlic, salt and pepper. Cook them (cut side down) for 10-15 minutes until crunchy.

Remove from oven, combine with nutritional yeast and add the yogurt on top.

Healthy tip: Do not overcook the Brussels sprouts as they lose nutritional value and will become bitter, with a sulfur smell. For optimal health benefits, consume fresh or lightly cooked/steamed cruciferous vegetables (such as Brussels sprouts, broccoli, kale and cabbage) two to three times a week.

Week 4 – Sunday

Gluten-Free Pancakes with Ricotta and Nuts
vegetarian-friendly

Servings: 2

Cook time: 20 minutes

Ingredients:

    1 cup buckwheat flour

    1 tablespoon baking powder

    1 cup milk

    1 + 1 teaspoons coconut oil

    ½ cup ricotta cheese

    1 teaspoon pesto

    ¼ cup pine nuts, roasted

Directions:

Preheat the oven at 425° F

In a bowl, combine the flour with baking powder. Add the milk, beaten egg, 1 teaspoon coconut oil and salt.

Place this mixture in a medium pan lightly coated with coconut oil. Bake until the pancakes are cooked through (15-20 minutes).

Cut into pieces, add pesto, ricotta and on top, the pine nuts.

> **Healthy tip:** The pancakes in this recipe are gluten-free. Coconut oil is recommended instead of butter. These can be served with fruits and yogurt as a dessert as well.

Homemade Buffalo Sauce

Ingredients:

- ½ teaspoon sweet paprika
- ½ teaspoon cayenne pepper
- 1 cup rice vinegar
- 2 cloves garlic
- 1 teaspoon olive oil
- Salt to taste

Directions: Place all the ingredients in a sauce pan over medium heat. Bring to a boil. Reduce the heat, cover and let simmer for 10 minutes. Place the mixture in a blender and blend until smooth.

Homemade Basil Pesto

Ingredients:

- 2 cups packed fresh basil leaves
- 2 cloves garlic
- ¼ cup pine nuts
- ⅔ cup extra-virgin olive oil, divided
- Salt to taste

Directions: Combine the basil, garlic, and pine nuts in a blender or food processor and pulse until coarsely chopped. Add ½ cup of the oil and continue processing until fully blended. Add salt to taste. Add cheese and all the remaining oil and pulse until smooth.

WEEK 4 SHOPPING LIST:

- One box quinoa
- One bag buckwheat flour
- One bag almond flour
- One bag/bunch baby spinach
- 2 tomatoes
- 1 red bell pepper
- Olives
- One bunch kale
- One avocado
- One small bag carrots
- 2 zucchini
- 2 cans mixed beans
- One can black beans
- Tomato paste
- One cauliflower
- 2 limes
- 1 lb Brussels sprouts
- One small bag pecans
- One small bag garlic
- One small bag onions
- Chili powder
- Baking powder
- Sweet paprika
- Cayenne pepper
- Pesto
- Eggs & egg whites
- Feta cheese
- Nutritional yeast
- 2 small yogurts
- Ricotta cheese
- Milk
- One bag corn chips
- Vegetarian hot dogs
- Olive oil
- Coconut oil
- One bottle rice vinegar
- Salt
- Pepper

Why Gluten-Free?

The wonderful thing about the recipes presented in this chapter is not just that they're nutritionally balanced, and not just that they present healthier alter- natives to unhealthy foods that you love. **The recipes are also gluten-free.**

And why is this important? Data on a study published by the National Institutes of Health (NIH) supports the benefits of gluten-free diets in reducing adiposity (fat) gain, inflammation and insulin resistance. Gluten-free animals showed a reduction in body weight gain and adiposity, without changes in food intake. The data further suggests that gluten-free diets should be considered as a new dietary approach to prevent the development of obesity and metabolic disorders.[5]

Is it any wonder that gluten-free menu items are now being made available at many restaurants and even fast food eateries? McDonald's, Cheesecake Factory, Taco Bell, Burger King, Wendy's, Olive Garden, P.F. Chang's, Baja Fresh, and almost everywhere you dine.

---

[5] *J Nutr Biochem, 2013 Jun;4(6):1105-11. doi: 10.1016/j.jnutbio. 2012.08.00. Epub 2012 Dec 17. Gluten-free diet reduces adiposity, inflammation and insulin resistance associated with the induction of PPAR-alpha and PPAR-gamma expression. Soares FL, de Oliveira Matoso R, Teixeira LG, Menezes Z, Pereira SS, Alves AC, Batista NV, de Faria AM, Cara DC, Ferreira AV, Alvarez-Leite JI.*

Healthy Snacks

On the Pound-a-Day Rapid Weight Loss™ program, you're not likely to get hungry in the mid-morning or mid-afternoon. But in the unlikely event that you crave something to munch on, here are some healthy snacks that are satisfying, and yet will help keep your weight under control:

A cup of berries

Apple (+ peanut or almond butter), or unsweetened apple puree

Popcorn (preferably air-popped and without butter – real or artificial). Avoid microwaveable popcorn. *Tip*: *Quinoa and amaranth also can be popped.*)

Kale chips

Corn chips (baked)

Carrot French fries

Baby carrots

Celery sticks

Oatmeal

Yogurt

Pumpkin seeds

A small handful of almonds, any other nuts and seeds, figs, raisins, edamame (soy beans)

Whey protein shakes (vegan formulas available)

Healthy tip: Always have a healthy snack available (but out of sight), whether you're on the go or at home or work. It can be your go-to food when you feel hungry, to avoid overeating or eating unhealthy foods.

Chocolate: A Healthy Snack That Can Help Make You Thin?

Chocolate is widely regarded as one of the most highly craved snacks, loved for its taste, scent and texture. But because of its high fat and sugar content, chocolate has always been demonized, regarded as an unhealthy food, and blamed as a major risk factor for obesity. Sugar-free chocolates, on the other hand, usually don't taste very good, but there's one exception.

Choco Perfection was voted the No. 1 Best-Tasting Sugar-Free Chocolate, and I concur. It is a guilt-free dark chocolate bar that tastes great, reduces sugar cravings, and actually supports weight loss because it uses oligofructose, a fiber-based sweetener, and none of the maltitol, an inferior sugar alternative that spikes insulin. The creator of these bars, Mary Jo Kringas, lost 75 pounds by eating 3 of these chocolate bars a day. See [*Recommended Websites and Resources* for more information.]

Chapter Six
Your Green Smoothie Recipes

Since green smoothies are such an integral part of the Pound-a-Day Rapid Weight Loss program, seven days' worth of healthy green smoothie recipes are presented in this chapter. These will help you get started on this healthy (and delicious) facet of the Pound-a-Day Rapid Weight Loss program.

You can also try your hand at creating your own recipes using this simple formula:

> 60% fruits (fresh or frozen)
>
> 40% green leafy vegetables
>
> 1 cup liquid (e.g., water, almond milk, coconut water)
>
> = 1 serving

To boost the nutritional content of your smoothie, add 1 scoop of a nutrient-dense superfood powder blend. (See *Recommended Websites and Resources* for a list of the best superfood powders that are widely available and resonably priced.)

Monday

Banana Mango Spinach Smoothie

Servings: 2

Ingredients:

- 1 orange
- 1 teaspoon lime juice
- 1 cup baby spinach
- 1½ cup sliced mango (fresh or frozen)
- 1 small banana
- 2 celery sticks sliced
- 2 cups water

Directions:

1. Combine the orange, 2 cups water, baby spinach, celery sticks mango and banana in a blender and puree until smooth.
2. You can add more water to reach the desired consistency.

> **Healthy tip:** Vitamins and minerals work synergistically, and one micronutrient can help better absorb other micronutrients. For example, iron from spinach will be better absorbed and utilized by the body when combined with vitamin C-rich foods such as orange, lime and mango.

Tuesday

Vanilla Berry Smoothie

Servings: 2

Ingredients:

> 1 cup raspberries (fresh or frozen)
> 1 apple
> ½ banana
> 1 kale (stems removed)
> 1 cup vanilla almond milk and 1 cup water

Directions:

1. Combine the raspberries, apple, almond milk, water, kale and banana in a blender and puree until smooth.
2. You can add more almond milk to reach the desired consistency.

> **Healthy tip:** Almond milk is a great alternative to cows' milk. It has fewer calories and carbohydrates. The same way iron needs vitamin C for better absorption, selenium works better when taken together with Vitamin E. Almond milk provides a healthy balance of vitamin E and selenium, as well as magnesium and manganese.

Wednesday

Beet Smoothie

Servings: 2

Ingredients:

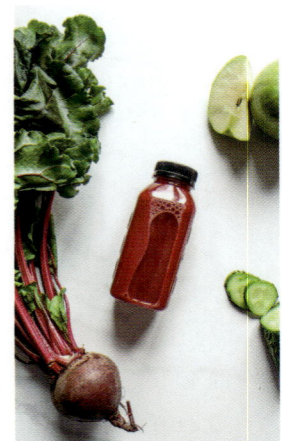

1 small beet (washed, peeled and chopped, fresh)

1 cup pineapple diced

1 small orange peeled

½ banana

1 kale (stems removed)

2 cups water

Directions:

1. Combine the beet, pineapple, water, kale and banana in a blender and puree until smooth.
2. You can add more water to reach the desired consistency.

Healthy tip: Fresh beets are rich in many healthy nutrients, including betalains—phytonutrients with strong antioxidant, anti-inflammatory and detox qualities.

Thursday

Avocado Peach Smoothie

Servings: 2

Ingredients:

- 2 cups peaches, sliced
- 1 medium avocado
- 2 tablespoons micro-milled chia seeds
- 1 kale (stems removed)
- 1 apple
- ¼ cup dates
- 2 cups water

Directions:

1. Combine peaches, avocado, flaxseeds, apple, kale, dates and water in blender and puree until smooth.
2. You can add more water to reach the desired consistency.

Healthy tip: An avocado has two times as much potassium as a banana. While your body needs this mineral for optimal health, don't overuse potassium-rich foods. You may want to try new recipes, but avoid combining an avocado and a banana in one smoothie—use one or the other, but not both. Chia seeds have been added to boost omega-3 fatty acids, and since avocado has more omega-6, this recipe has a good balance between these omega fatty acids.

Friday

Pomegranate Kiwi Smoothie

Servings: 2

Ingredients:

    1 cup pomegranate seeds

    5 kiwi fruits, peeled

    1 cup mango

    2 tablespoons of micro-milled chia seeds

    ½ cup baby spinach

    ½ cup romaine lettuce

    2 cups water

Directions:

1. Combine the pomegranate seeds (ok if some pith still attacked to the seeds), kiwis , flaxseeds, mango, spinach, lettuce and water in a blender and puree until smooth.
2. You can add more water to reach the desired consistency.

Healthy tip: Pomegranate has antioxidant qualities superior to cranberries and even green tea. It is rich in polyphenols, anthocyanins, as well as vitamins C, K, and folate. It also helps optimize cholesterol levels and aids weight loss.

Saturday

Sunflower Smoothie

Servings: 2

Ingredients:

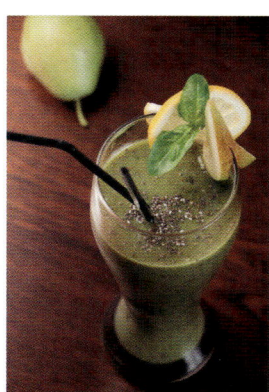

- 1 orange
- 1 apple
- 1 banana
- 1 cup chopped raw sunflower seed sprouts
- 2 cups water
- Optional: 1 tablespoon fresh parsley leaves

Directions:

1. Combine the sunflower green sprouts (remove the hulls), orange, apple, banana, (parsley optional) and water in a blender and puree until smooth.
2. You can add more water to reach the desired consistency.

Healthy tip: Sprouts are incredibly nutritious, and can be 10 times (or more) richer in nutrients compared to the original seed from which the sprout originates. They're also easier to digest since they contain enzymes that make the digestion easier. This is why they are also known as "pre-digested foods." Use them quickly after removing them from the pot, as they start losing vitamin content within an hour.

Sunday

Collard Green Smoothie

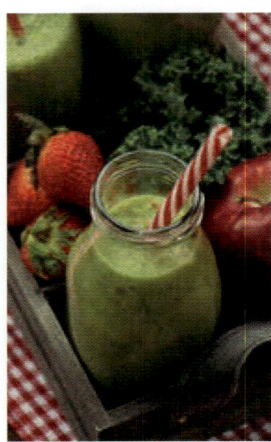

Servings: 2

Ingredients:

    2 cups of collard greens – stems removed

    1 peach

    1 cup blueberries

    1 medium carrot, chopped

    1 cup coconut water & 1 cup water

    1 teaspoon coconut oil (optional)

Directions:

1. Combine the collard greens, carrot, peach, blueberries, water, coconut water (+/- coconut oil) in a blender and puree until smooth.
2. You can add more coconut water to reach the desired consistency.

Healthy tip: Collard greens are less bitter than kale or dandelion greens, but packed with vitamins and minerals (especially high in vitamin K). Collard greens are flavorful, and help you lose weight faster.

One-Week Shopping List
FOR SMOOTHIES ONLY

3 bananas (also buy extra bananas for snacks)

3 apples (also buy extra apples for snacks)

3 oranges (also buy extras for snacks)

3 limes

2-3 mangoes

1 pineapple

3 peaches

1-2 pomegranates

1 box fresh raspberries

1 box fresh blueberries

1 small box dates

5 kiwis

1 avocado

1 bag celery sticks

1 bunch collard greens

1 bunch kale

1 bag baby spinach

1 small bunch beets

1 bag romaine lettuce (hearts)

1 pot sunflower seed sprouts

Vanilla almond milk (unsweetened)

1 bag Pound-a-Day Rapid Weight Loss micro-milled chia seeds

1 bottle coconut water

1 jar of coconut oil

Optional: one bunch fresh parsley

Chapter Seven
The 1-Minute Mindset Technique

Scientifically "rewire your brain" to get rid of food cravings, compulsive eating habits and emotional factors that are obstacles to losing weight

Imagine yourself being hungry ... and craving a burger, a pizza, or a slice of cake. What if you could tap a few points on your head and upper body – and suddenly, in as little as a minute or two, you no longer had the food craving?

How much weight could you lose with this magical power – and how happy would that make you feel?

Now, imagine yourself feeling lonely, stressed out, bored, or just tired after a bad day at work. And all you want to do is sit in front of the TV and devour a bag of potato chips ... or a box of chocolate chip cookies ... or a pint of ice cream ... or whatever comfort food you can find in your kitchen. What if you simply tapped a few parts of your head and upper body – and suddenly, **the need for binge eating disappeared into thin air**?

With this super power, how likely would it be for you to lose weight rapidly – and keep the weight off permanently? Very likely indeed! In fact, **it would be almost impossible to fail**.

The Pound-a-Day 1-Minute Mindset Technique™ (hereinafter referred to as the Mindset Technique) is based on the scientifically validated healing modality called Emotional Freedom Technique, which is also called "tapping." The Mindset Technique was designed to be used in conjunction with the Pound-a-Day Rapid Weight Loss program.

<u>Here's how the system works</u>: The Pound-a-Day Rapid Weight Loss program provides **the structure through which you can shed weight easily** – with no meal plan or restrictive diet, and no counting calories, no measuring food, and no counting points – just 5 of the most effective weight loss strategies rolled into one powerful plan that optimizes your health while enabling you to lose weight.

The Mindset Technique is the indispensable tool you can use to support your weight loss efforts and enables you to stick to a healthy lifestyle, thereby helping you lose excess weight—*even when nothing else seems to work*. Without the Mindset Technique, there is a high likelihood that you will fail to lose weight permanently because of the hidden reasons that sabotage your weight loss efforts.

Scientifically Validated to Rewire Your Brain in Minutes

The Mindset Technique is a simple healing modality that combines the power of acupressure, energy medicine and modern psychology. This technique involves gently tapping energy meridians in your body with your fingertips, accompanied by positive affirmations that, together, send a calming signal to the part of the brain called the amygdala.

The energy meridians are the same ones used in traditional acupuncture to treat physical and emotional ailments – but without the use of needles.

This combination of tapping the energy meridians and voicing positive affirmations rewires your brain by reprogramming your limiting patterns, beliefs and negative traumas – and releasing emotional blocks.

Compared to psychotherapy, which is slow and cumbersome when it comes to creating mental, emotional and psychological change, this technique rewires your unconscious brain – **fast**.

The Mindset Technique virtually eliminates 99% of those hidden reasons, pitfalls and obstacles that could potentially get in the way of your weight loss success – *without requiring you to use willpower*.

When you learn this simple technique, it will enable you to ...

- "turn off" your food cravings at will;
- eliminate emotional eating, which is responsible for approximately 75% of all weight gain;
- reduce your body's levels of the stress hormone (cortisol), which makes you gain weight;

- overcome negative beliefs, emotions and thought patterns – and replace them with positive thoughts and feelings; and
- rewire your brain to defuse the negative programming that makes you unconsciously sabotage your weight loss efforts.

Widely renowned and respected integrative physician, Dr. Joseph Mercola, uses this healing modality to help patients overcome negative emotions. "We also use it to reduce food cravings that can sabotage healthy eating programs," he states, "and to implement positive life goals to support optimal health and well-being."

The Mindset Technique can be learned by anyone quickly and easily in just a few minutes – and you can apply the technique on yourself in the comfort of your own home, or wherever you are. And, as its name suggests, it can be done in only 1 minute or less.

In the section of this chapter titled *How to Do the 1-Minute Mindset Technique*, there is a link to an online video that will demonstrate step-by step how to do this technique. By the time you try it a few times, you'll be a master of the technique – and well on your way to ultimate weight loss success with the Pound-a-Day Rapid Weight Loss program.

As simple as the Mindset Technique may seem, there's an abundance of scientific evidence of its efficacy. More than 50 researchers in 7 countries have carefully studied the tapping technique – including prestigious institutions, such as Harvard Medical School, the University of California at Berkeley, Johns Hopkins, Texas A&M, and the Walter Reed Army Medical Center. Their findings have been published in more than 15 different peer-reviewed journals.

Because of its very high rate of success, the practice of tapping has spread rapidly – and medical practitioners employing this technique are now commonplace in every part of the world. Quite simply, it works!

Once you learn the Mindset Technique for facilitating permanent weight loss, it can also be used to improve many other areas of your life. Numerous clinical studies on this technique have produced impressive results in the following applications:

- Elimination of pain—including fibromyalgia and seizure disorders
- Alleviating anxiety, depression and emotional challenges—including the reduction of public speaking anxiety, psychological trauma in veterans, long-term psychological symptoms, test anxiety in university students
- Getting rid of phobias and addictions

- Enhancing athletic performance
- Neutralizing Post-Traumatic Stress Disorder (PTSD)

The tapping technique has also been used to overcome insomnia, break out of emotional gridlock, improve athletic performance, and eliminate limiting beliefs that prevent you from creating fruitful relationships or achieving financial success.

Why You Must Learn the 1-Minute Mindset Technique Before You Start the Pound-a-Day Rapid Weight Loss Program

Without the proper mindset and emotional balance, all weight loss efforts are doomed to fail – or weight loss success will be temporary, at best. But when you possess the proper mindset and emotional balance, it's almost impossible to fail in efforts to lose weight permanently. This is what makes the Mindset Technique an essential adjunct to the Pound-a-Day Rapid Weight Loss program.

There are 3 primary reasons why you must learn and practice the Mindset Technique as soon as you can:

1. Overcome the Mental, Emotional and Psychological Reasons for Weight Gain

One of the major reasons why most people fail to keep the weight they lost from coming back is because most weight loss programs address only the PHYSICAL mechanisms of weight loss ... such as reducing calories, carbohydrates and fat ... boosting metabolism ... and exercise. They ignore the MENTAL, EMOTIONAL and PSYCHOLOGICAL reasons for weight gain.

Our brains are programmed – or "wired"– with deeply ingrained attitudes ... preconceived notions ... and programmed beliefs that cause us to behave in ways that are sometimes counterproductive to our weight loss goals. These include ...

- Low self-esteem
- Fear of failure
- Fear of not being good enough
- Perfectionism
- Need for control
- Self-doubt

- Anger issues
- Need for acceptance

When we harbor these programmed beliefs, attitudes and feelings, what do we do?

We eat.

We also eat as a means of coping with our emotions. We eat when we're sad ... when we're angry ... when we're tired ... when we've had a bad day ... when we're feeling lonely or heartbroken ... when we're bored ... when we've been rejected – or when we're experiencing stress.

We eat ... and then we eat some more ... mistakenly thinking that food will fill the void, the emptiness, the feelings of self-loathing that fill our day-to-day existence.

And we eat even when we're not hungry. This is what is called **emotional eating**.

Emotional eating accounts for an estimated 75% of all weight gain, according to Jane Jakubczak, RD, LD, dietitian at the University of Maryland in College Park

Face it. There's a high likelihood that you will succumb to emotional eating frequently during any of your attempts to lose weight. So you need the Mindset Technique as a tool to help you overcome your tendency to eat as a way of coping with emotions.

And you also need the Mindset Technique to put a stop to food cravings and overcome the limiting beliefs and negative programming that keep the excess weight from being shed permanently.

Relying on will power simply <u>won't</u> work. <u>Case in point</u>: In 2002, the *Today* show's Al Roker lost more than 100 pounds after undergoing gastric bypass surgery. But in less than 5 years, he had regained much of the weight. He described his struggle in a TV interview, stating that he began to regain the weight when his mother was ill in the hospital. Because he worried so much about his mother's welfare, his old eating habits came creeping back and he turned to junk food to cope. Roker's experience shows us that will power simply cannot overcome our fixation on food when we're emotionally overwhelmed. Al Roker's inability to keep the weight off does not mean he lacks self-control, willpower or the strength to do whatever it takes to keep the weight off. It just means he's human, just like you and me.

We all fall prey to the temptation of binge eating when we need something – anything – to help numb our emotional pain and negative programming.

Food is – and always has been – the most convenient and readily available coping mechanism for most people. It's no wonder why one-third of the American population – and a significant percentage of the rest of the world – is overweight.

With the Mindset Technique, you now have a simple 1-minute mechanism you can employ so that you'll never need to turn to food to fill the void or the emptiness.

Whenever you think you're hungry, ask yourself the question: "What am I really hungry for?"

More often than not, what you're feeling is not real hunger, which is your body needing nourishment. You're feeling empty and hungry for something else such as love, social connection, balance and purpose.

And yet, even when you do realize what you're really hungry for, you still reach for food because it's an easy fix -- instant gratification.

Practical Application: Whenever you have a desire to binge eat ... or you think you're hungry but realize you're really hungry for something else other than food ... or you experience specific food cravings ... you can do the Mindset Technique instead of reaching for food. You'll find that after doing the technique for a minute or two, the "artificial" hunger would have disappeared.

[See section in this chapter titled **How to Do the 1-Minute Mindset Technique** to view the online video demonstrating step-by step how to do this technique.]

2. Eliminate Stress-Induced Weight Gain

Your body produces a hormone called cortisol as a result of being exposed to stress. When the body senses danger – whether real or imagined – such as a stressful situation or fearful thoughts – it goes into a physiological state called the fight-or-flight response. This response causes the body's energy to be diverted towards self-preservation or self-defense, and causes the production of excessive amounts of cortisol, also referred to as the stress hormone.

Studies have shown conclusively that high levels of cortisol are linked to increased appetite, an overabundance of abdominal fat, and sugar cravings.

If the body's exposure to stress is only occasional, this wouldn't be a matter of serious concern. But because the average person lives with stress on a daily basis, the overproduction of cortisol slowly but surely causes you to gain fat and weight, and makes it difficult to shed unwanted weight.

Even though you may have think you have a healthy lifestyle – you're eating a balanced diet, and you're exercising regularly – the presence of too much stress-induced cortisol in your body may well be the reason why your weight just won't budge.

Dawson Church, Ph.D, a widely recognized expert on energy psychology, and a master practitioner of EFT (or tapping) on which the Mindset Technique is based, conducted a study that produce significant results. Dr. Church's randomized controlled study set out to determine how tapping would impact the cortisol levels of 83 subjects compared to the cortisol levels of people who received traditional talk therapy, and the cortisol levels of those who received no treatment at all.

The results were both significant and compelling. Those who underwent a tapping session experienced an average cortisol reduction of 24% to 50%. Those in the other 2 groups (traditional talk therapy or no treatment at all) did not experience any significant cortisol reduction.

Eliminating excess cortisol alone could single-handedly account for tremendous weight loss. This is why the Mindset Technique could potentially make a significant difference in your weight loss efforts.

Practical Application: Whenever you are experiencing stress – whether mild or severe – do 2 repetitions or more of the Mindset Technique. This will send a calming signal to the amygdala of the brain, and help prevent the production of excess cortisol in your body.

[See section titled **How to Do the 1-Minute Mindset Technique** to view the online video demonstrating step-by step how to do this technique.]

3. Reverse Engineer Your Weight Loss: Don't Put Your Happiness on Hold

If you're like most people who struggle with excess weight, you have the tendency to put your life on hold until you've lost all your unwanted weight. You put aside doing the things you would love to do until that day that you've achieved your ideal weight. And you put your happiness in limbo and wait for that fateful day to arrive.

What you may not know is that living in limbo in this way is the surefire way to not lose the weight – and not achieve your ultimate purpose for wanting to lose weight in the first place. The author Carnelian Sage conveyed this message so simply, but profoundly, as follows:

> "Consider why a person would want to lose weight – usually it's because they want to look good. Why do they want to look good? Because they want to gain the approval or admiration of others – or themselves. When you break their motives down further, you arrive at the one core reason why they do what they do. It's because deep down, what they truly want is love. They want other people to love them – and they want to love themselves." – Excerpt from *The Greatest Manifestation Principle in the World* by Carnelian Sage

And there you have it – the most fundamental of all human needs. Loving and accepting one's self is at the core of all endeavors, whether it be weight loss or any other endeavor. The only reason you wish to lose weight is because you think you can find happiness outside of yourself – usually through the approval of other people.

Your self-talk goes something like this: "If I lose weight, then I'll feel proud of myself, then I'll love myself and be happy."

Therefore, if your ultimate goal for wanting to lose weight is to love yourself, then you can "reverse engineer" the weight loss journey by starting at the end – love yourself first.

On the surface, this might seem like stating the obvious because who, after all, doesn't love themselves? You'd be surprised. One shouldn't confuse self-centeredness and selfishness as being the same as loving one's self. Loving yourself means deeply and completely accepting yourself ... taking responsibility for your own needs and feelings, being complete in and of yourself, and acknowledging an internal source for all your needs instead of looking to external sources (people, places and things, including food) to fill your needs.

An amazing thing happens when you deeply and completely accept and love yourself ... you spontaneously behave in ways that enable you to naturally lose excess weight, automatically get rid of food addictions and mental obsessions – and rise above any and all human dilemmas

Practical Application: Whenever you are experiencing bouts of self-loathing or low self-esteem ... or you're struggling with body image dissatisfaction (body hating) ... or suffering from obsessive perfectionism – do 2 or 3 repetitions of the Mindset Technique. This will enable you to eliminate the shame and bondage associated with excess weight, replace self-loathing with self-love, silence the negative self-talk in your brain, and help you develop a healthy body confidence

[See section titled **How to Do the 1-Minute Mindset Technique** to view the online video demonstrating step-by step how to do this technique.]

How to Do the Pound-a-Day 1-Minute Mindset Technique

The basic technique of the Mindset Technique is simple and easy – and takes only a few minutes to learn. It involves 3 things: Focusing on the issue to be resolved—whether it be stress, negative emotions, food cravings, body image dissatisfaction, or low self-esteem—while simultaneously tapping on certain areas of the head, face and body and voicing affirmations.

Go to www.Pound-a-Day.com/MindsetTechniqueVideo.mp4 for a step-by-step video demonstration.

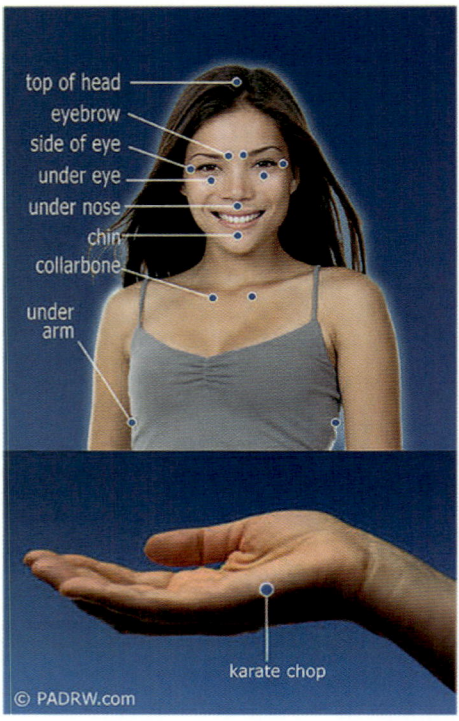

Tapping Points: You will be tapping your fingers on the energy meridians listed below (and pictured above):

>   Top of the head
>   Inner Eyebrow (near the bridge of the nose)
>   Outside corner of the eye (on the bone)
>   Under the eye (on the bone)
>   Under the nose
>   Chin
>   Collarbone
>   Under the arm (about 4 inches below the armpit)

It's important to tap the correct area, but you need not worry about being overly precise with pin-point accuracy. Tapping the general area is sufficient.

You may tap with the fingers of the right hand (or the left, if you're left-handed). There are meridian tapping points located symmetrically on either side of the body, so it won't matter which side you tap.

You should tap firmly, but never so hard as to hurt yourself. And tap with your fingertips, if you can, but if you have long nails, you can use your finger pads.

You will tap on each tapping point about 5-7 times, or about the same length of time as one full breath. One cycle of tapping all points will take approximately one minute – hence, the name The 1-Minute Mindset Technique.

Note: Remove your eyeglasses or watch prior to practicing the Mindset Technique since these items may mechanically and electromagnetically interfere with the effects of the technique. [Go to www.Pound-a-Day.com/MindsetTechniqueVideo.mp4 for a step-by-step video demonstration.]

Tuning In to the Problem You Want to Resolve: Rate the Intensity on a Scale of 1 to 10

Tuning in to the problem at hand (such as a food craving, stress, negative emotion, or other problem you want to resolve) is an important part of the Mindset Technique.

Here's why: The cause of all negative emotions is a disruption in the body's energy system. When you are tuned in to the problem, it causes your energy system to disrupt, and consequently brings about negative emotions. Without tuning in to the problem, there is no energy disruption that the Mindset Technique can seek to balance.

Tuning in to a problem can be done by simply thinking about the problem and how it makes you feel. Thinking about the problem will bring about the energy disruptions. The Mindset Technique can then clear the "short-circuit" – the emotional block – from your body's energy system, thus restoring your mind and body's balance.

For example: If the problem you wish to resolve is stress, tune in to how you're feeling. When you tune in (or listen to what your body is saying about the stress), you may be able to recognize the stress as a knot in your stomach, or a heaviness in your chest, or shallow breathing, a sore neck or a headache. Really tune in to how the stress is making you feel and rate it on a scale of 1 to 10, with 10 meaning an extremely high stress level, and zero meaning you're completely relaxed with not a care in the world.

[Go to http://www.Pound-a-Day.com/MindsetTechniqueVideo.mp4 for a step-by-step video demonstration.]

What to Say While Tapping

Now that you're acquainted with the tapping points, how to do the tapping, and how to tune in to the problem you're trying to resolve, you will next need to know what to say while you are tapping.

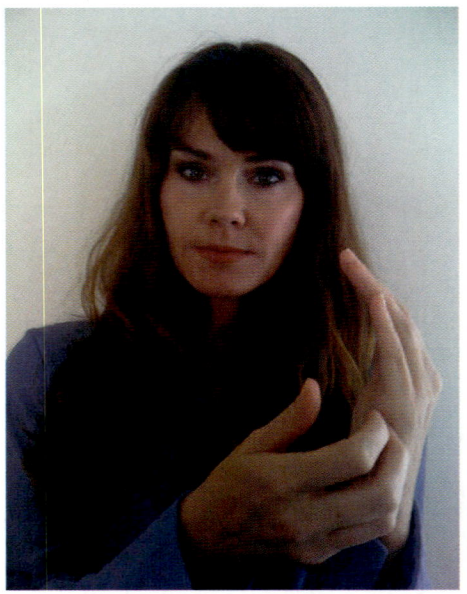

A) The Setup Statement that you should use while tapping the karate chop point of your hand (which is the same setup statement used in traditional tapping or EFT) is as follows:

"Even though I have this _____, I deeply and completely accept and love myself."

You fill in the blank above with a brief description of the stress, food craving, negative emotion, body image dissatisfaction, or other problem you want to resolve.

Sample setup statements you can use: The following examples represent a variety of problems related to weight management, but you can tailor them your setup statement to suit the specific problem you have.

"Even though I'm feeling so stressed about my weight, I deeply and completely accept and love myself."

"Even though I have all this stress, and my stomach is in knots, I deeply and completely accept and love myself."

"Even though I'm feeling stress about my finances and my job, I deeply and completely accept and love myself."

"Even though I have this craving for ice cream (or pizza, potato chips, or cake), I deeply and completely accept and love myself."

"Even though I don't like how I look in the mirror, I deeply and completely accept and love myself."

"Even though I have this anger towards my boss, I deeply and completely accept and love myself."

"Even though I have this memory of physical abuse, I deeply and completely accept and love myself."

"Even though I sometimes feel I'm not good enough, I deeply and completely accept and love myself."

"Even though I have these nightmares, I deeply and completely accept and love myself."

"Even though I have an inferiority complex, I deeply and completely accept and love myself."

"Even though I'm deeply hurt and heartbroken, I deeply and completely accept and love myself."

[Go to http://www.Pound-a-Day.com/MindsetTechniqueVideo.mp4 for a step-by-step video demonstration.]

B) After saying the Setup Statement while tapping on the karate chop point, proceed tapping all the 8 tapping points in succession – while continuing to tune in to how the problem is making you feel, and saying affirmations, thoughts and feelings you have about your problem.

For example: If you're tapping to resolve a problem with stress, these are the words you could say while tapping on the 8 tapping points:

"This stress in my body."

"This stress is intense."

"I feel this stress in my chest (or my head, neck, shoulders, as the case may be)."

"This stress feels overwhelming."

"This stress feels out of control."

"I love and accept myself, and I'm open to releasing these emotions."

"I feel the stress in my body. My chest is heavy and my breathing is shallow."

"I'm allowing my body to feel calm."

"Releasing the stress in my body."

"Allowing my body to feel calm and relaxed."

"Infusing my body with joy, love and peace, regardless of the stress in my life."

"My stomach is feeling calmer, more relaxed."

"As I let go, my whole body feels calmer."

"My body feels calmer and relaxed as I release and let go."

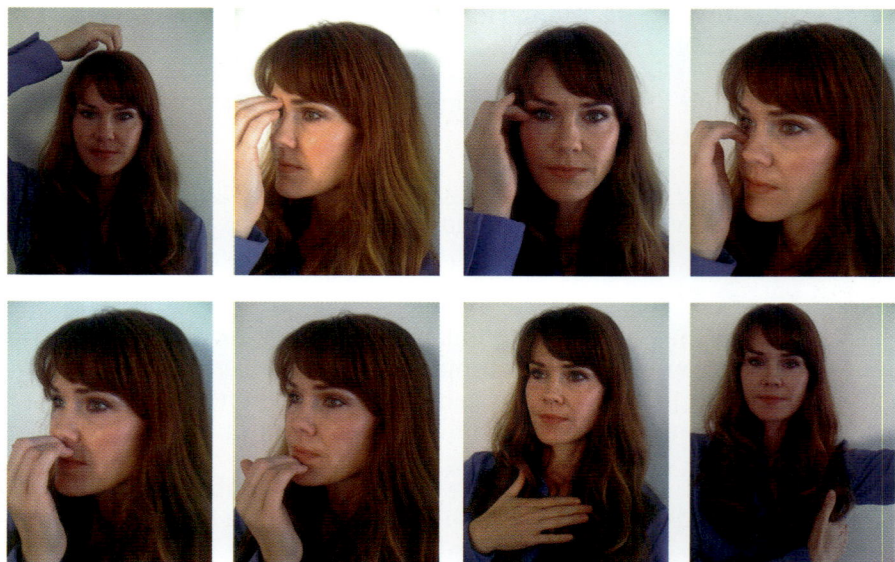

Take a Deep Breath and Rate the Intensity of the Problem Again

After tapping on the karate chop point (while saying the setup statement described in Section A); and after tapping on all 8 tapping points (while saying the suggested affirmations described in Section B); repeat the entire cycle 1 or 2 times; and end the session by taking a deep breath and exhaling.

Now, tune in to how you're feeling after your Mindset Technique session. Did it come down to a lower number compared to the rate you gave prior to the session? Did it come down to zero?

Really tune in to what that feels like to know that your emotions – and all the repercussions of emotions – are under your control with the Mindset Technique. And if you still feel like there's still a bit of the problem remaining (and sometimes there might be because you must get very specific about how you're feeling), then you may choose to do a few more sessions of tapping one more round of tapping.

USEFUL TIPS:

- Just say the setup statement or affirmations, whether you believe them or not. Not believing them won't diminish the effectiveness of the Mindset Technique.
- If you can say the setup statement or affirmations with conviction and feeling, that would be ideal. However, if you initially cannot, saying them repeatedly will often do the trick.
- Whenever possible, say the setup statement or affirmation aloud.

However, if you're unable to, you may whisper it under your breath, or do it silently.

When to Use the 1-Minute Mindset Technique to Empower Your Weight Loss Efforts

After you've learned how to do the Mindset Technique, you can use it as often as you want during the day to empower your weight loss efforts on the Pound-a-Day program.

Remember, it's your most powerful tool for overcoming 99% of the hidden reasons, pitfalls and obstacles that could potentially get in the way of your weight loss success. It is a scientifically validated solution that enables you to achieve permanent weight loss—even when nothing else has worked before.

Following are the best times during the day when you can do the 1-Minute Mindset Technique:

◆ **In the morning, upon waking up**

Body image dissatisfaction and feelings of low self-esteem and defeat over weight loss failures often start the moment you wake up. You may find that you often indulge in negative self-talk in the morning, such as "I'm so fat" or "I hate how I look" or "I'm stressed out even thinking of trying to lose weight."

Therefore, the best way to start your day is to eliminate the negative emotions by doing 2 or 3 rounds of the Mindset Technique, which significantly helps erase your negative self-talk, enhances body confidence, and gives you a sense of empowerment and control.

Suggested setup statements:

"Even though I hate how my body looks, I deeply and completely accept and love myself"

"Even though I'm stressed out about trying to lose weight, I deeply and completely accept and love myself."

◆ **Whenever you have food cravings**

Ninety-seven percent of women and 67% percent of men experience food cravings – that intense yearning for specific foods that are usually unhealthy and fattening. Some people crave sugary food like chocolates, cake and ice cream; others crave rich, fat-laden, and greasy foods like burgers, fries, or fish and chips; and others crave high-carb or salty foods like pizza, pasta or potato chips.

Clearly, giving in to your food cravings frequently will lead to an overconsumption of calories and, consequently, weight gain. So whenever you're faced with a food craving, do 2 or 3 rounds of the Mindset Technique to reduce the likelihood of indulging in that craving – without having to use will power.

Suggested setup statement:

"Even though I crave ice cream (or pizza, or cake, or potato chips, as the case may be), I deeply and completely accept and love myself."

♦ **Whenever you're tempted to give in to emotional eating**

As previously mentioned, emotional eating is responsible for approximately 75% of all weight gain. So whenever you're lonely, heartbroken, having a bad day, feeling rejected, tired, bored, or feeling other emotions that make you want to eat when you're not hungry, do 2 or 3 rounds of the Mindset Technique to satisfy what your body really wants – a calming of those intense emotions, not food.

Suggested setup statement:

"Even though I'm depressed (or lonely, heartbroken, having a bad day, feeling rejected, tired, or bored, as the case may be), I deeply and completely accept and love myself."

♦ **Whenever you're experiencing stress**

Statistics from a recent global stress research study show that stress is prevalent worldwide. Everyone experiences stress occasionally or frequently in all spheres of life. We stress out about demands or problems at home, work, school, and personal relationships. A recent survey shows that the #1 stress among adult women involves their weight.

As mentioned in the previous section, stress causes the production of excessive amounts of cortisol, also referred to as the stress hormone. High levels of cortisol are linked to increased appetite, an overabundance of abdominal fat, and sugar cravings – and therefore, contributes significantly to weight gain, no matter how devoted you are to a healthy lifestyle, diet and exercise.

Therefore, to prevent stress from sabotaging your weight loss efforts, whenever you're feeling stress during the day, do 2 or 3 rounds of the Mindset Technique. The Mindset Technique will send a calming signal to the part of your brain called the amygdala, clear any emotional blocks from your energy system, and restore balance to your mind and body. More importantly, the Mindset Technique will reduce cortisol production in your body significantly, which will greatly contribute to weight loss.

- **Whenever you want to overcome your negative programming that sabotages your weight loss efforts**

    Whether you realize it or not, there are negative beliefs, emotions, habits, traumas and thought patterns that have been programmed in your brain for years (sometimes since early childhood), which make you unconsciously sabotage your attempts to lose weight.

    For example, you may have been told by your parents to eat everything on your plate because there are so many starving children in the world. Or you might have adopted your family's habit of eating potato chips, sugary treats or unhealthy snacks while watching TV. Or you might have learned to use food as a "reward" for doing a good job. Or you might have acquired the common habit of using food as a way to cope with your problems. Or maybe you might have had a traumatic experience that continually wreaks havoc on your eating habits.

    Whatever your negative programming may be, you can neutralize it by doing 2 or 3 rounds of the Mindset Technique anytime during the day. Doing the Mindset Technique will rewire your brain by reprogramming your limiting patterns, beliefs and negative traumas – and releasing emotional blocks.

    Suggested setup statements:

"Even though I have this urge to eat everything on my plate, I deeply and completely accept and love myself."

"Even though, my father abandoned me when I was little, I deeply and completely accept and love myself."

"Even though I have this memory from my childhood (specify the memory, if applicable), I deeply and completely accept and love myself."

"Even though I'm tempted to eat a bag of potato chips while watching TV, I deeply and completely accept and love myself."

"Even though I'm worried that my father (or husband, wife, friend or loved one, as the case may be) is sick, I deeply and completely accept and love myself."

"Even though I'm going through a difficult time in my life, I deeply and completely accept and love myself."

Using the 1-Minute Mindset Technique with the Pound- a-Day Rapid Weight Loss Program

The 1-Minute Mindset Technique, used on its own, will help tremendously in eliminating your food cravings and emotional eating – and rewiring your brain with a mindset that puts you on the road to a healthy lifestyle. But you still need to have some kind of structure in your life if you want to get rid of the 10, 30, 50 pounds or more of excess weight. That weight took years to accumulate in your body – and it won't miraculously disappear just because you rewired your brain.

The 1-Minute Mindset Technique was designed to work hand in hand with the Pound-a-Day Rapid Weight Loss program, which works with your body's biochemistry – and makes it appear that excess weight automatically falls off, as if on cue. To recap, the program combines the 5 most effective strategies for losing up to a pound a day, and is the only program that ...

- allows you to eat your favorite food (no meal plan or restrictive diet)
- doesn't require you to count calories or measure the amount of food you consume
- is so simple and easy to follow that you'll want to stick to it ... for life!
- enables you to lose weight – but more importantly, keep the weight off effortlessly, supported by your healthy lifestyle and the 1-minute mindset technique

When you use the 1-Minute Mindset Technique together with the Pound-a-Day Rapid Weight Loss program, you can accelerate your weight loss and finally keep the weight off ... forever.

Chapter Eight
The 20-Second Workout

The minimum effective dose of exercise which will give you a lean, firm, toned and metabolically efficient body

When it comes to evaluating the merits of thousands of different fitness programs currently available, there is simply no comparison: Programs based on High-Intensity Interval Training (HIIT) come out ahead on many different fronts. But when it comes to choosing among various types of HIIT exercise routines, the **20-Second Workout (20SW)** described and demonstrated in the pages of this chapter stands head and shoulders above the rest, for two reasons.

The first has to do with the exercises themselves. The 20SW program employs exercises that utilize the **minimum effective dose** of exercise you can do -- and still see results. And that minimum effective dose is **20 seconds**.

That's because it takes as little as 20 seconds per muscle group to experience a change in your physique. When you engage one muscle group with a 20-second high-intensity contraction, your body gets the signal that it needs that muscle, so it will then hold on to it -- making the body more metabolically efficient -- instead of letting that muscle tissue waste away.

But the REAL SECRET is that unlike standard isolated exercises which target a specific set of muscles, the **20-Second Workout (20SW)** is comprised almost exclusively of compound exercises. Compound exercises target a broad range of muscle groups simultaneously, which means they are super time-savers. After all, why spend hours and hours exercising when you can achieve the same—or better—results in minutes? That would be like making multiple trips to the grocery store and buying a single item each time, rather than just making one trip and getting everything you need at once.

The 20-Second Workout (20SW) enables you to shape up and tone your whole body quickly -- and achieve the same (or better) results than hours of standard cardio or aerobic exercises.

Best of all, the compound exercises of the 20SW are supported by scientific studies that show that they contribute to cardiovascular health ... make the body more metabolically efficient ... optimize the loss of unwanted weight ... stimulate muscle development ... promote faster calorie burn (which means significantly increased fat loss) ... enhance coordination and joint stability ... and minimize the risk of injury.

The exercises that comprise the 20-Second Workout are a perfect complement to the weight you will lose on the *Pound-a-Day Rapid Weight Loss* program. After all, who wants to simply lose weight and not have a lean, toned, firm and well-defined body?

The 20-Second Workout has been carefully designed with two goals in mind: to help you fulfill your fitness goals; and to make your fitness routine fit as seamlessly as possibly into your busy lifestyle so that it's easy to maintain.

Compound exercises alone already put the 20SW far ahead of most other HIIT programs. But it also includes a strong focus on *plyometrics*, a class of exercises that super-charge your body's ability to **burn the maximum number of calories in the shortest amount of time**. In essence, plyometrics (also known as "jump training") are designed to cause muscles to move from an extended state to a contracted state as quickly as possible, so that the muscle exerts an explosive burst of maximum force.

Sprinting, high jumping, and depth jumping (off a platform) are all types of plyometric exercise. Because they help increase muscle strength, they are often used by professional athletes to help improve speed, power, and overall performance.

In fact, Russian athletes training for the Olympics have been using plyometrics since the 1960s, when they were developed by Dr. Y. Verkhoshansky.

Another factor that makes the 20SW superior to other HIIT programs is that it uses the optimal ratio of exercise to rest, which is 2:1 (20 seconds exercise: 10 seconds recovery), as endorsed by top fitness experts.

~~~~~

In the following pages, you'll find descriptions and images for all the exercises included in the 20SW. There's also a link next to each exercise which leads to an online video demonstrating the correct way to do the exercise in order to achieve optimum results.

Before you begin, though, there are a few guidelines that will help you work out effectively and safely.

[1] Talk to your doctor before beginning any HIIT workout in order to determine the suitability of these exercises for your particular fitness level and assess any factors that might indicate a risk for you.

[2] If you experience chest discomfort or any other symptoms during your workout, stop immediately, and seek medical advice.

[3] If you are unable to jump, you can skip the parts of the following exercises that include jumping. If the reason you can't jump is due to an ankle or knee injury, I don't recommend that you do any of the pylometrics exercises at all, but feel free to modify the rest to meet your needs.

[4] Monitor your heart rate. One easy way to do this is with a heart watch monitor. Another method is to use a stop watch, and ensure that your heart rate stays at 90% of your maximum heart rate for cardio exercises, and 70-80% for the rest. The formula provided by the American Heart Association for determining your maximum heart rate is 220 minus your age. So if you are 40 years old, your maximum heart rate would be 180.

[5] If you are taking medication for high blood pressure, be aware that some of these types of medications can lower your maximum heart rate.

[6] Don't try to do too much too soon. Take your cue in this respect from babies, who learn to sit, crawl, stand, and walk before they are ready to run and jump. Adapt the exercises to your fitness level.

[7] When you're starting out, technique is much more important than speed. Take the time to learn the exercises properly before you worry about doing them quickly. Speed will come with practice and familiarity. Warming up before your workout and cooling down afterwards are important not only to make your work out more effective, but also to prevent injuries.

[8] Although you need minimal equipment for the 20SW routine, I do suggest that you purchase a tape measure so that you can keep track of your progress. Don't forget to measure (waist, hips, and thighs) before your first workout, so you can compare where you started to your ongoing progress.

[9] Follow the 20SW formula as closely as you can. Remember, this means working out 4 times a week, as follows:

Three times a week:

10 exercises (20 seconds each); each exercise is followed by 10 seconds of recovery time

10 X 30 seconds = **5 minutes** [choose any 10 exercises from the list below for this workout]

Once a week:

4 exercises (20 seconds each); follow each exercise with 10 seconds of recovery time, followed by 10 seconds of recovery (time: 30 seconds X 4 = 2 minutes)

4 X 30 seconds = 2 minutes [choose *any* 4 plyometrics exercises for this workout]

If you're interested in working on your triceps, exercise #11 is one of the best! Add it to your workouts as a bonus, bringing your total workout time to 5½ minutes.

And of course, if you'd like to speed up your results even faster, you can always double the duration of your workout, so you're doing 4 minutes once a week, and 11 minutes three times a week. However, refrain from doing a plyometrics workout more than twice a week.

Work at the Proper Intensity

You will need to work out at a 9 to 9.5 intensity level (90% - 95% of you max heart rate) for your cardio and plyo exercises in order to burn fat. All other exercises can be done at an intensity of 80%.

Choosing Your Exercises

Below you'll find detailed descriptions for all exercises, along with images and links to online video so you'll know exactly how to perform each one.

Warm-Up Exercises

Before exercising it is very important to warm up the muscles, ligaments and tendons to prevent injuries and muscle soreness. Warming up also helps prepare the nervous and cardiovascular systems. As such, dynamic exercises, such as jogging in place, walking lunges, and squats performed for 30 seconds and then repeated for a further 30 are much better for warm-ups than slow, yoga movements.

Cool-Down Exercises

Cooling down after exercise reduces muscle stiffness and soreness because it helps your body flush out the waste products (lactic acid) accumulated during your workout. For this purpose, static, gentle exercises work best, because they help slow your heart rate, decrease blood pressure and body temperature, and improve flexibility. The following exercises are all excellent for cooling down.

The 20-Second Workout Exercise List

1. Bear crawl

For killer abs, and strong, lean thighs and shoulders

Target: Abs, Butt/Hips, Legs/Thighs, Shoulders, Full Body/Integrated

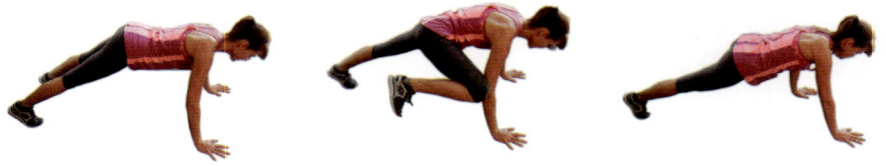

For a video demonstration of this exercise, go to
https://www.pound-a-day.com/20swvideodemos/#BearCrawl

- From a push up position (hands and feet wide apart), walk your left hand and right foot forward at the same time

- Return to starting position, then repeat the movement right hand and left foot

- Keep your abdominal muscles tight , so your spine will be straight and the pelvis stable during the workout

- If you have limited space you can move forward and backward as needed, but continue to move and do so as quickly as you can

2. Donkey kicks

Great butt-beautifying potential

Target: Abs, Butt / Hips

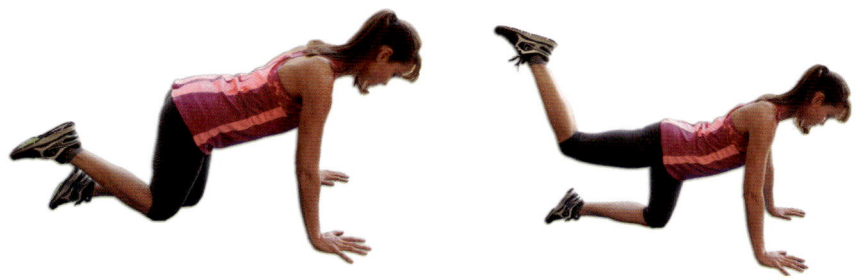

For a video demonstration of this exercise, go to
https://www.pound-a-day.com/20swvideodemos/#DonkeyKicks

- Start from the quadruped position (hands and knees on the floor, with your knees and feet hip –width apart and your hands under your shoulders). Keep your spine straight and in a neutral position by keeping your abdomen muscles tight

- Lift the left leg and bend the knee at 90 degrees. Contract your glutei (butt) muscle and press the foot toward the ceiling (move only the hip joint, do not move the knee joint)

- Lift the leg until the heel of the foot is pointing toward the ceiling and the leg is lined up with the body; repeat for 10 seconds, then switch legs and perform repeats for 10 seconds with the right leg for 10 seconds with the left leg, switch the legs and perform reps for 10 seconds with the right leg.

Along with squats, this exercise is ranked as most effective for tightening your butt, and it's one of the few isolated exercises that will give you quick results in a short period of time.

3. Squats

Another super butt-beautifier

Target: Abs, Butt, Hips, Calves and Shins, Thighs

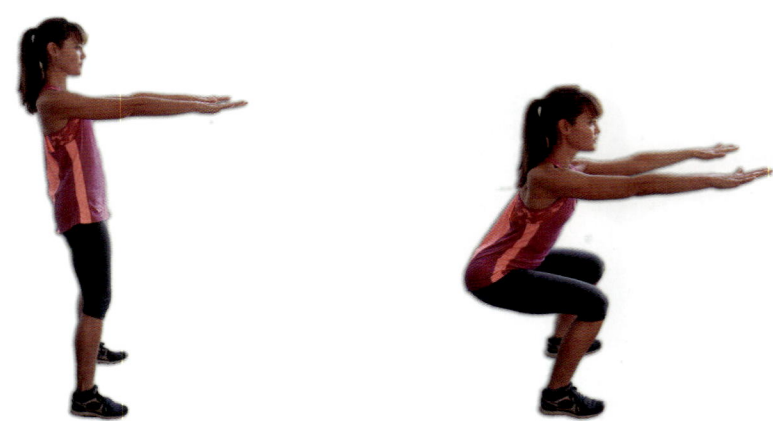

For a video demonstration of this exercise, go to
https://www.pound-a-day.com/20swvideodemos/#Squats

- Stand with your feet hip-distance apart, toes pointed straight forward

- Tighten up your abs, lift your chest up tall while pulling the shoulder blades back and down during the entire exercise

- Keeping the chest up, sit back as far as you can (as if you are going to sit in a chair)

- Keep the knees over the ankles (do not push them forward over the toes)

- When you are in this position, bring your thighs parallel with the floor

- Repeat as fast as you can for 20 seconds

4. Side Lunge:

Shapes the butt, sheds the inner thigh fat, improves balance and hip flexibility

Target: Butt/Hips, Inner and Outer Thighs

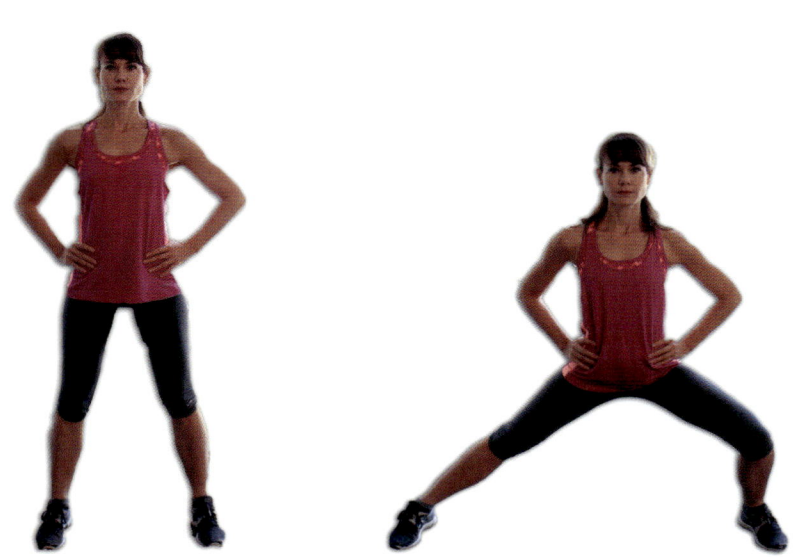

For a video demonstration of this exercise, go to
https://www.pound-a-day.com/20swvideodemos/#SideLunge

- Stand with your feet hip-width apart, hands on your hips

- Keep your chest up tall and proud, while pulling your shoulder blades back and down during the entire exercise; Toes should be facing front

- Take a big step to the side with your left leg, bend your left knee, and push hips back and down(so the left knee is bent 90 degrees)

- Push back to starting position, repeat the movement for a total of 10 seconds, then repeat with your right leg for the remaining 10 seconds

5. Knee Drivers

Choice of professional runners; increases speed and power

Target: Thighs, Butt/ Hips

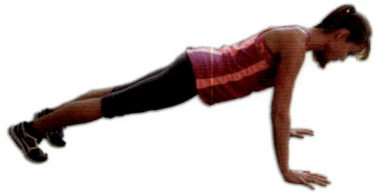 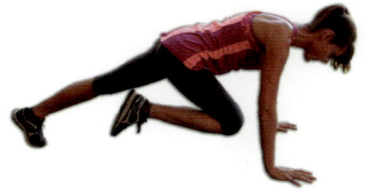

For a video demonstration of this exercise, go to
https://www.pound-a-day.com/20swvideodemos/#KneeDrivers

- Start the exercise in a push up position; keep your arms straight and hands below the shoulders

- Take right foot off the floor and bring the right knee into your chest

- Return to starting position, than take the left foot off the floor and bring it to the chest

- Repeat, alternating legs, for 20 seconds without pausing

6. Jab and Cross

No more flabby arms!

Target: Arms, chest, shoulders, core

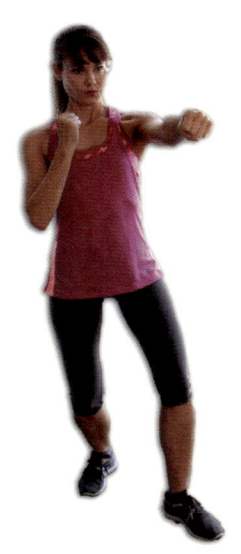 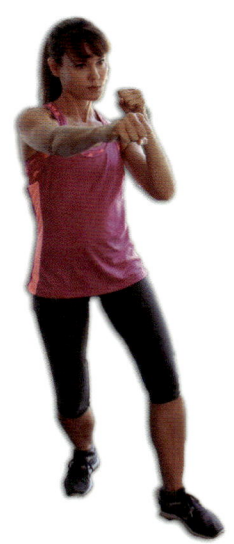

For a video demonstration of this exercise, go to
https://www.pound-a-day.com/20swvideodemos/#JabAndCross

- From an on-guard position (right foot forward, elbows bent, hands curled into fists on either side of your chin) throw a quick jab (punch) with your right arm, while rotating your fist down; do not lock your elbow.
- Follow with a quick left cross (punch your left arm forward, rotating your left hip into the punch and lifting your left heel off the floor
- Bring your arms back to on guard position and repeat
- Keep the core (abdominal muscles) tight during the entire workout
- Speed is very important

7. Glute Kicks

Butt-kicking calorie burner

Target: Butt / hips and thighs

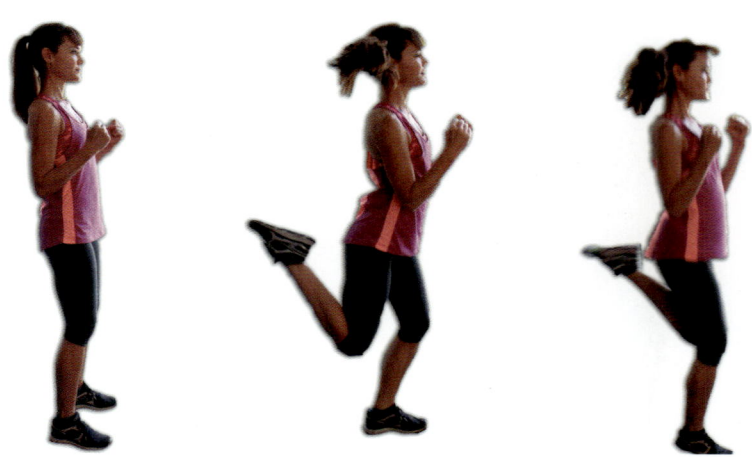

For a video demonstration of this exercise, go to
https://www.pound-a-day.com/20swvideodemos/#GluteKicks

- Stand with feet close together and knees slightly bent, with your heels hip-width apart. Bend your elbows, keeping your hands close to the body

- Kick your right foot up and back, so that the heel touches the right gluteus muscle (the butt). Your right thigh should be almost perpendicular to the floor.

- Switch, kicking your left heel up to your left gluteus (left butt)

- Repeat for 30 seconds, as quickly as you can.

Don't worry if you can't touch the butt with your foot at the beginning; as your fitness level improves, you will be able to accomplish this.

8. Single Dumbbell Swings

Sleek, sexy arms in no time; great for core and lower body, too.

Target: Arms, shoulder, butt, thighs, core

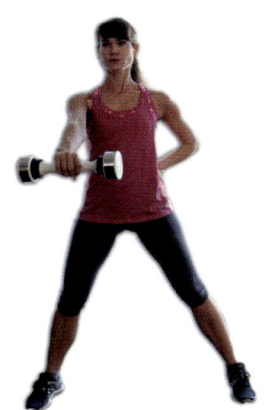 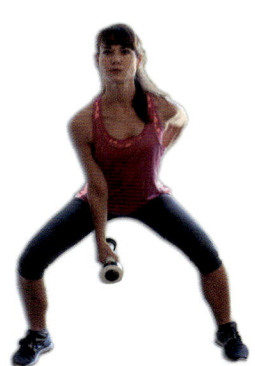

For a video demonstration of this exercise, go to
https://www.pound-a-day.com/20swvideodemos/#SingleDumbbellSwings

For this exercise you can use dumbbells if you wish, but you can also use items you already have around the house (2 full cans of food; 2 water bottles or milk jugs filled with sand or water). The key idea is to use something with a bit of weight to it, and that you can comfortably hold in your hand. If you are working on improving your strength, work with heavier weights and do fewer repetitions; if you are focusing on building endurance, use a lighter weight and more repetitions.

- Place your feet 2-3 feet apart and hold a weight in your right hand (palm facing downward)
- Squat down until your thighs are almost parallel to the floor, and move the weight between your legs
- Thrust your hips forward, straighten your knees, and swing the weight up to chest level, keeping your arm straight
- Squat back down, swing the weight between your legs, and you are done with your first rep
- Repeat with your other arm.
- Keep your core (abdominal muscles) tight at all times

9. Lunge & Twist

The magic is all in the twist!

Target: Core, butt/hips, thighs

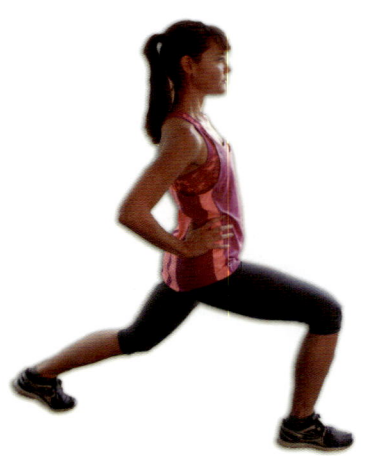 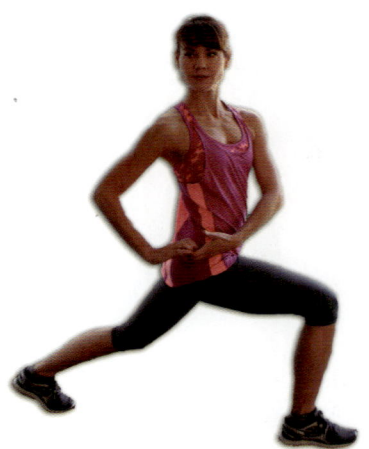

For a video demonstration of this exercise, go to
https://www.pound-a-day.com/20swvideodemos/#LungeAndTwist

- Stand with feet together
- Bring right foot forward and lunge
- Hold at the bottom of the lunge and twist slightly towards the left side
- Repeat on opposite side
- Do as many reps as you can for 20 seconds
- If you need to hold on to something for balance (example: a chair) you may do so.

This is a great exercise to improve balance and stability. It's vastly better than regular lunges, because while the lunging motion isolates and shapes your quads and hamstrings nicely, the twist helps your glutes to contract more while the core is also engaged.

10. Superman / Superwoman

Fabulous for back and butt

Target: Core (great for lower back), butt, thighs

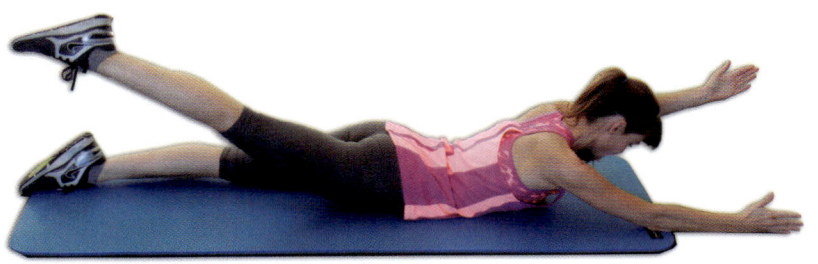

For a video demonstration of this exercise, go to
https://www.pound-a-day.com/20swvideodemos/#Superman

- Lie on the floor on your stomach with your arms extended straight forward (over your head, as if you are reaching for something), and your legs straight and front of feet touching the floor

- As you exhale, squeeze the muscles of your back so that your left arm and right leg raise off the floor [this is a small, controlled movement focused on contracting the back muscles]

- Return to the starting position, and repeat with your right arm and left leg

11. Bicycle Crunch

Show off your 6-pack!

Target: Core

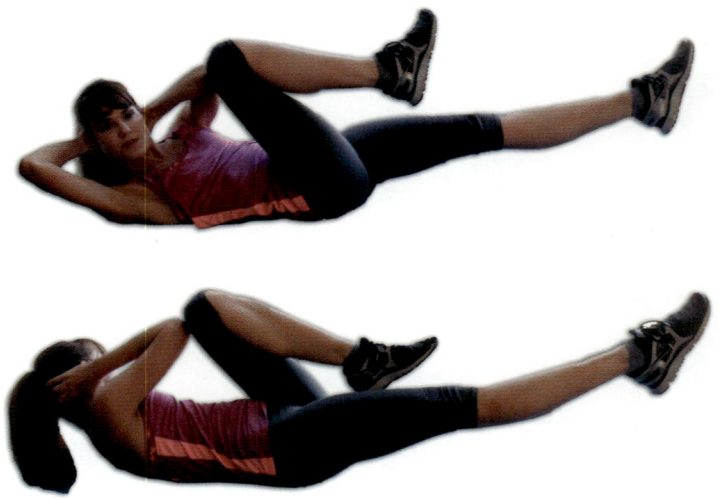

For a video demonstration of this exercise, go to
https://www.pound-a-day.com/20swvideodemos/#BicycleCrunch

- Lie flat on the floor, keeping your lower back pressed to the floor
- Contract your core muscles
- Holding your head with your hands, lift your knees to about a 45-degree angle and perform a bicycle pedaling motion, while alternately touching each elbow to the opposite knee
- Do as many reps as you can for 20 seconds

BONUS EXERCISE: Tricep Dip!

Target: Triceps/ the arms, chest, legs

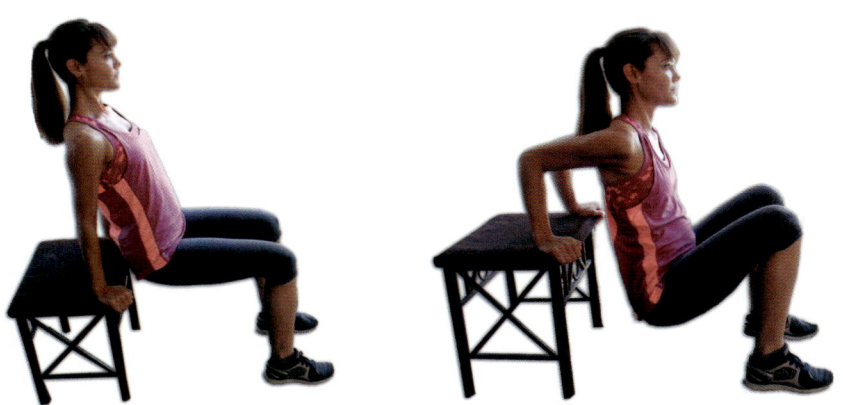

For a video demonstration of this exercise, go to
https://www.pound-a-day.com/20swvideodemos/#TricepDips

- Sit on the edge of a low bench or a sturdy chair, knees bent, feet flat on the floor

- Place your hands, palms facing down, on either side of the hips with fingers extended over the edge, arms straight. Scoot forward on the bench until your hips and butt are in front of the seat

- Bend your elbows so that the hips drop below the level of the bench, and arms are parallel to the floor

- Push back and start another rep

- Do reps for 20 seconds

Exercises Part II: PLYOMETRICS

1. Chair Pose

For fabulous legs and strong core

Target: Butt, legs, shoulders, and back

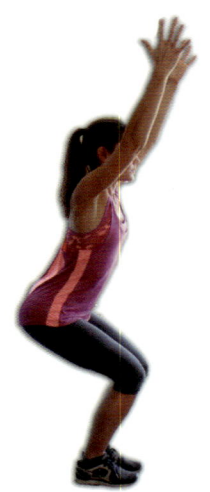 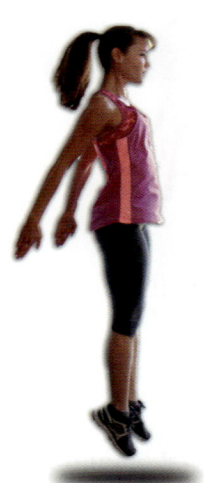

For a video demonstration of this exercise, go to
https://www.pound-a-day.com/20swvideodemos/#ChairPose

- Stand straight, feet together, arms straight at your sides with the palms facing your thighs
- Squat and at the same time, raise your arms over your head
- Jump up out of the squat, bringing the arms down to your sides and then out behind you
- Swing arms forward to your sides so you land in the same position your started

Non-plyo version: Skip the jump and simply squat and rise up, following the same arm movements.

2. Burpees

Belly be Gone!

Target: Thighs, legs, core

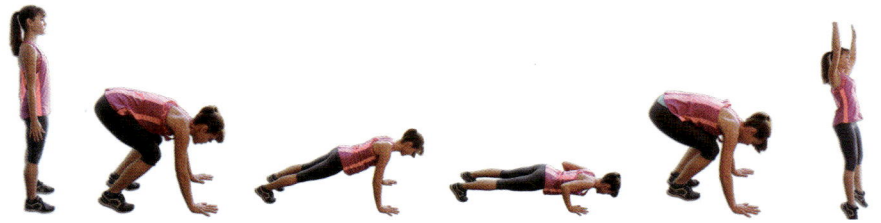

For a video demonstration of this exercise, go to
https://www.pound-a-day.com/20swvideodemos/#Burpees

- Stand up tall, feet shoulder-width apart
- Bend your knees, place your hands on the floor
- Jump your feet out behind you so that they are straight and you land in a push-up position
- Keeping your hips in line with your shoulders quickly hop your feet back in and stand up, keeping your weight on your heels and your back straight

Non-plyo option: Skip the jumping and complete a modified burpee by squatting down, walking your legs out straight behind you (one by one) then stepping them forward again into a squat, then stand up.

3. Plyo Broad Jump

For a beach body

Target: Butt, legs, core

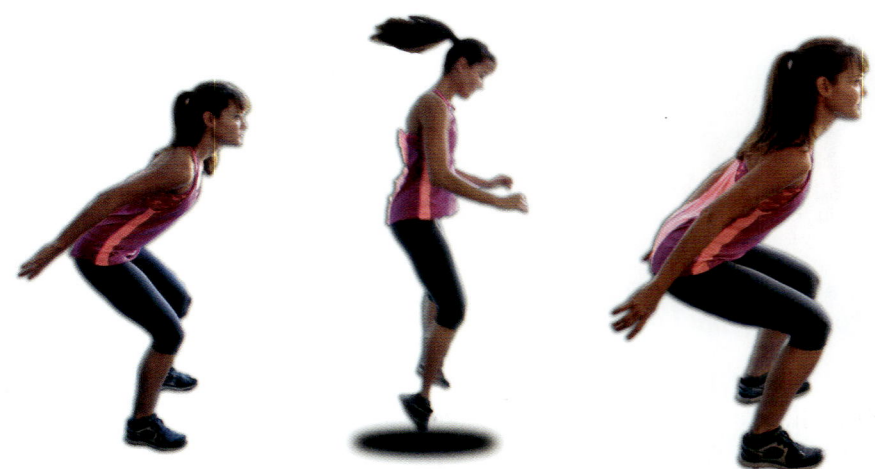

For a video demonstration of this exercise, go to
https://www.pound-a-day.com/20swvideodemos/#BroadJump

- Stand with your feet hip width- apart

- Drop into a squat with your weight on your heels (your knees should be over your toes) keeping the back flat

- Leap forward as far as you can, throwing your arms forward to start the movement

- Land on your feet in a bent-knee position (weight on your heels)

- As you touch the ground, quickly leap forward again in the same manner

Variations: Decrease your jump distance to make it easier; or simply turn it into a squat. But keep in mind that the further you jump, the more muscles you work, so try to jump as far as you can on each repetition.

4. Plyo Jab, Cross and Squat

For sleek, sexy arms and a flat belly

Target: Arms, butt, legs, core/whole body

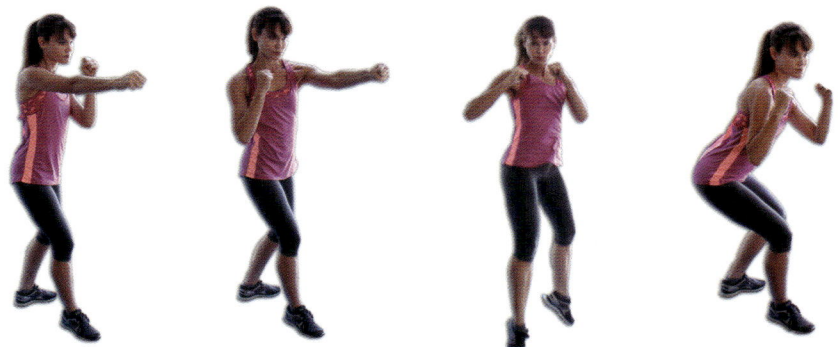

For a video demonstration of this exercise, go to
https://www.pound-a-day.com/20swvideodemos/#PlyoJabCrosAndSquat

- From an on-guard position (right foot forward, elbows bent, hands curled into fists on either side of your chin) throw a quick jab (punch) with your right arm, while rotating your fist down; do not lock your elbow.

- Follow with a quick left cross (punch your left arm forward, rotating your left hip into the punch and lifting your left heel off the floor

- Perform 2 quick punches

- Bring your arms back to the on guard position

- Quickly push your hips back and lower into a squat

- Jump up, land and get into the on-guard position and repeat with the opposite arm

- Keep the core (abdominal muscles) tight during the entire workout

- Speed is very important so do this sequence as quickly as you can

Non-plyo version: Skip the jump and the squat.

5. Plyo Lateral Ankle Hops

For shapely legs and ankles

Target: Legs (including inner thighs) butt, core With dumbbells: Arms

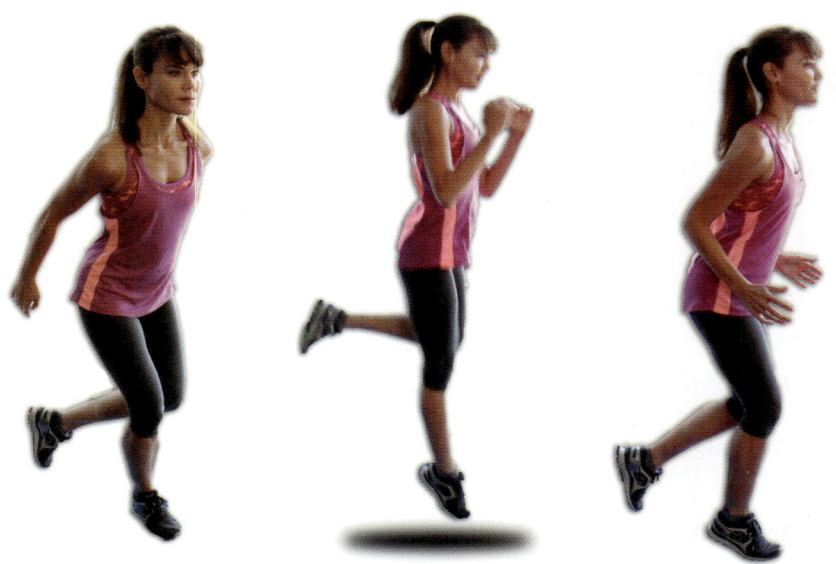

For a video demonstration of this exercise, go to
https://www.pound-a-day.com/20swvideodemos/#LateralAnkleHops

- Stand straight with your feet apart
- Bring your left leg up, knee bent
- Hop to your right, landing on your right foot
- Quickly switch, bringing your right leg up and hopping to your left. This is one rep of the exercise.
- Do as many reps as you can in 20 seconds

To make the exercise more difficult, increase the width and/or height of your jumps

Non-plyo option: Skip the hop.

6. Mountain Climbers

Target: Legs, butt, core, arms/ whole body workout

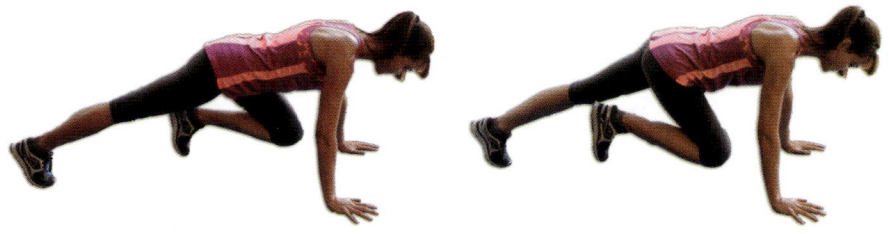

For a video demonstration of this exercise, go to
https://www.pound-a-day.com/20swvideodemos/#MountainClimmbers

- Start from a push-up position with your hands shoulder-width apart
- Bring the right knee in towards the chest
- Jump up and switch feet in the air, bringing the left foot to the chest and the right foot back. This is one rep.
- Do as many reps as you can in 20 seconds

Option: To make it easier, you can use a bench or other sturdy raised platform.

7. Mountain Climbers (with bench)

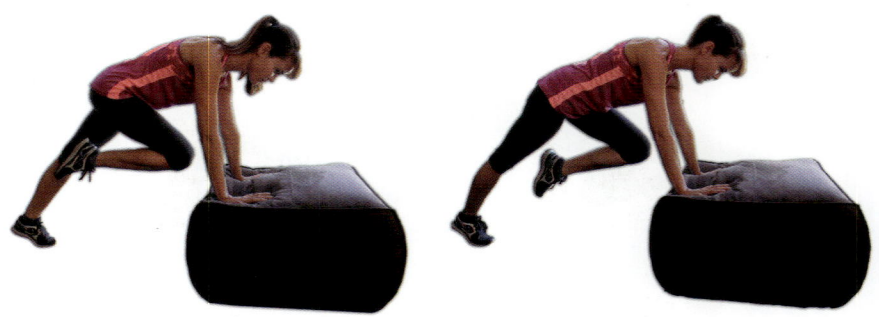

For a video demonstration of this exercise, go to
https://www.pound-a-day.com/20swvideodemos/#MountainClimbersWithPlatform

Option 2: Skip the jump and simply walk.

The steady running motion activates your glute and leg muscles; while your core muscles, including your back, hips and abs, will also work hard to maintain stability; shoulders and chest are also trimmed and toned. The closer you keep the hips on the floor, the stronger you will get.

Non-pylo option: Skip the jump and walk instead of running.

8. High Knees

Natural enemy of belly fat

Target: Butt, legs, core, cardio

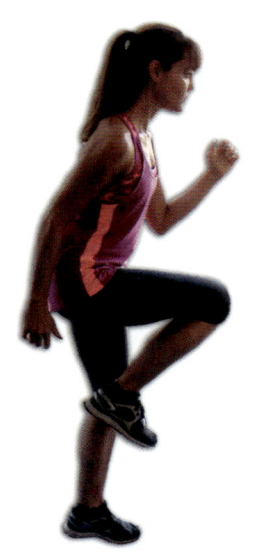 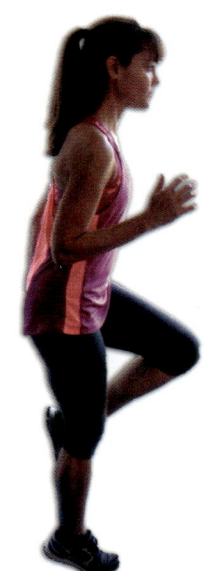

For a video demonstration of this exercise, go to
https://www.pound-a-day.com/20swvideodemos/#HighKnees

- Keeping your upper body straight, start running in place
- Keep your left knee high (the higher the better) and swing your right hand
- Switch, and bring your right knee high, while swinging your left hand
- Repeat as fast as you can for 20 seconds

9. Rock Star Hops

Mega calorie burner

Target: Legs, butt, core / whole body

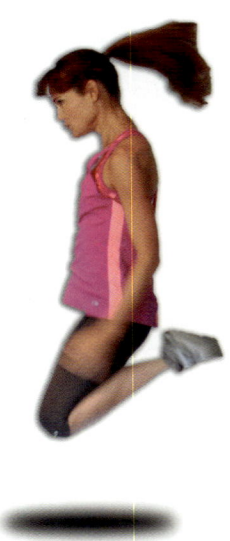 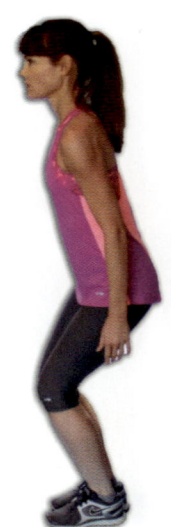

For a video demonstration of this exercise, go to
https://www.pound-a-day.com/20swvideodemos/#RockStarHops

- Stand with your feet shoulder-width apart
- Jump straight up as high as you can and try touching your heels to your butt.
- Land with your knees bent
- Quickly jump up again

Non-pylo option: Skip the jump, and bring one heel at a time to the butt.

10. Jumping Jacks

Target: Legs, butt, core, arms / full body workout

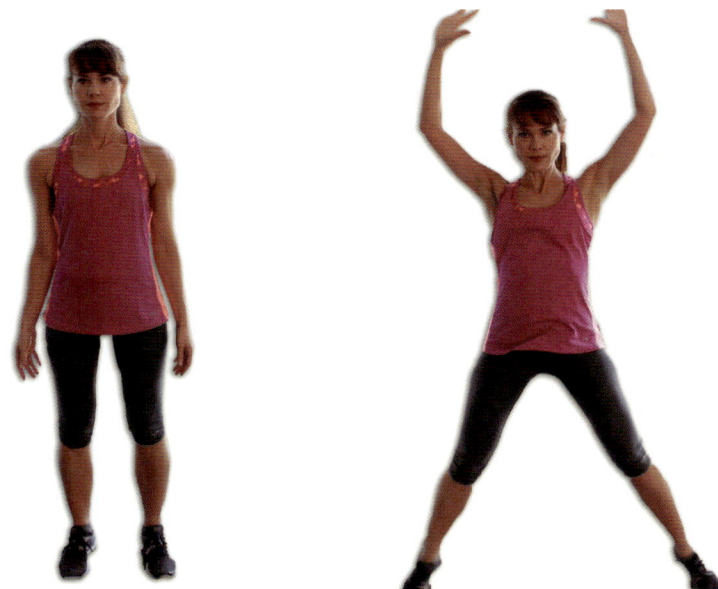

For a video demonstration of this exercise, go to
https://www.pound-a-day.com/20swvideodemos/#JumpingJacks

- Start with your feet hip-width apart and hands at your sides
- Raise both arms above your head and jump
- Repeat. Do as many reps as you can for 20 seconds

Hamstring Stretch

Stretch one leg out in front of you, keeping the knee straight. Bend the back leg slightly. Hands on hips, gently push the hips backwards and hold for 20 -30 seconds.

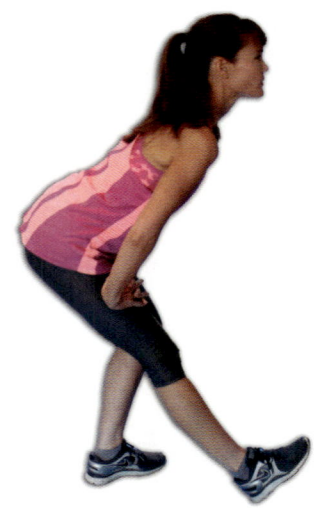

Quad Stretch

Balance on one leg, bend the other leg back and upwards (towards your butt). Reach back and grab your toes, pulling the heel in towards your butt. Keep your core strong and tight. Hold for 20-30 seconds.

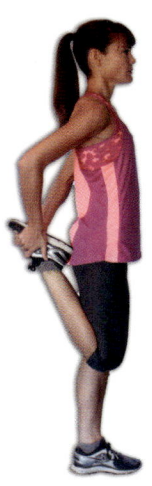

Chest Stretch

Clasp your hands behind your back and bring your shoulder blades down and closer together. Pull your elbows in toward each other as far as you can. Hold for 20-30 seconds.

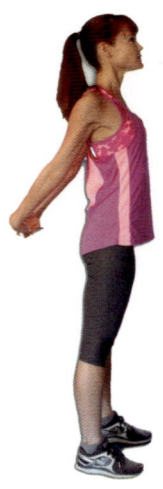

Upper Back Stretch

Bring your hands together in front of your body. Bring your chin close to the chest and push your hands forward. Hold for 20-30 seconds.

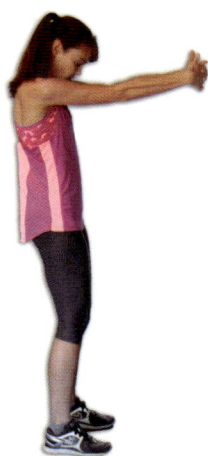

And there you have it, the 20SW exercises that will have you well on your way to your ideal fitness level ... 20 seconds at a time!

RECOMMENDED WEBSITES AND RESOURCES

The 3 supplements that are key to the effectiveness of the Pound-a-Day Rapid Weight Loss program (glucomannan capsules 2000mg, organic chia seeds and pu-erh tea), are all available online at www.OnePoundADay.com.

Other recommended brands for the 3 supplements:

Glucomannan:
Carlyle Glucomannan Capsules, 2400mg
Nova Nutritions Konjac Root Glucomannan Capsules, 2000 mg

Pu-Erh Tea:
Numi Organic Tea Emperor's Pu-erh Tea, 16 Count Tea Bags
Prince of Peace 100% Organic Pu-erh Tea, 100 Count Tea Bags

Organic Chia Seeds:
BetterBody Foods Organic Chia Seeds, 32 Oz
Sun Harvest Organic Chia Seeds, 16 Oz

Recommended Superfood Powder Supplements:

Garden of Life Raw Organic Perfect Food Green Superfood Juiced Greens Powder, 7.3 oz

Orgain Organic Superfoods with Probiotics, 0.62 pounds

Organifi Original Green Juice, 9.8 oz

Beyond Greens™ Energy, Detox & Immunity Mix, 0.25 pounds (4 oz)

Garden of Life Raw Organic Perfect Food Green Superfood

Enso Superfoods Supergreens, 8.5 oz

Choco Perfection – Voted the No. 1 Best-Tasting Sugar- Free Chocolate Bar (with no aspartame or artificial sweeteners) www.ChocoPerfection.com

Green Smoothie Phenomenon - This book reveals the single most health-enhancing, weight-reducing, healing, detoxifying and anti-aging habit for achieving optimum health—green smoothies! Includes 49 kitchen-tested recipes that enhance your health and well-being. www.GreenSmoothiePhenomenon.com

The One-Minute Cure: The Secret to Healing Virtually All Diseases – This book, which has been the No. 1 Amazon.com bestseller in the Health category more than 15 times, reveals the remarkable, scientifically proven natural therapy that creates an environment within the body where cancer and other diseases cannot thrive—and enables the body to cure itself of disease. www.1MinuteCure.com